FIGHT DISEASE WITH A POWERFUL SEED

Prevent & Reverse:

- Cancer
- Heart Disease
- Diabetes
- Alzheimer's and more!

The Wonders of French Grape Seed Extract

Terry Lemerond

and

Ajay Goel, Ph.D.; M.S.

The purpose of this book is to educate. It is not intended to serve as a replacement for professional medical advice. Any use of the information in this book is at the reader's discretion. This book is sold with the understanding that neither the publisher nor the author has any liability or responsibility for any injury caused or alleged to be caused directly or indirectly by the information contained in this book. While every effort has been made to ensure its accuracy, the book's contents should not be construed as medical advice. To obtain medical advice on your individual health needs, please consult a qualified health care practitioner.

Copyright © 2020 TTN Publishing, LLC. Green Bay, WI

www.TTNPublishing.com

All rights reserved. Any excerpts as permitted under the United States Copyright Act of 1976, no part of this publication in any format, electronic or physical, may be reproduced or distributed in any form or by any means or stored in a database or retrieval system without the prior written permission of the publisher.

Library of Congress Control Number: 2020911252

Print ISBN: 978-1-952507-04-5
eBook ISBN: 978-1-952507-01-4

Editor: Michele Olson
Design: Larry Bowers
Formatting: Alt 19 Creative

Printed in the United States of America

This book is dedicated to all the true health seekers in the world.

Contents

Part 1: French Grape Seed Extract Can Help You Beat Cancer 1
   1   Nature's Multi-Tasker 3
   2   A Powerful Natural Answer to Cancer..... 11
   3   A Shotgun Approach to Cancer 23
   4   Wipe Out Cancer Stem Cells 33
   5   The One-Two Punch...................... 41

Part 2: French Grape Seed Extract's Power Against Other Diseases....................... 49
   6   Insidious Inflammation and Obdurate Oxidation................................ 51
   7   A Guardian Against Heart Disease 61
   8   A Tool in the Fight Against Metabolic Syndrome, Type 2 Diabetes, and Obesity .. 71
   9   Stop the Memory Robber.................. 81
  10   A Powerhouse Against Other Diseases and Conditions............................... 89
  11   Know How to Find the Right Choice 95
  12   Doc to Doc 103
References 113

About the Authors.............................. 115
References 117
More about TTN Publishing, LLC................. 127
Welcome to TTN Publishing!..................... 128
Share this exciting news! 129

PART 1:
French Grape Seed Extract Can Help You Beat Cancer

CHAPTER 1
Nature's Multi-Tasker

Meet Mother Nature's multi-tasker. There are few botanicals, herbs, plants, or foods that have the humble grape plant's power—whose health benefits have elevated it to the rank of royalty in the plant world.

There are only a handful of botanicals known today that can achieve these remarkable healing feats:

- Reduce inflammation, an underlying factor in many chronic diseases
- Prevent and treat cancer by attacking it in several ways
- Lower blood pressure
- Strengthen and relax blood vessel walls
- Lower cholesterol and triglycerides
- Control blood sugars
- Help you lose weight
- Protect brain cells
- Protect memory by helping create neural pathways as alternative pathways to transmit information

As a cancer researcher, Dr. Goel is certainly impressed with this range of healthful benefits, and especially with the cutting-edge research his team has completed that confirms its powerful activity against the deadliest cancers.

What is This Royal Botanical?

French grape seed comes from the royalty of grapes. Think of French wine, and you'll quickly get the idea. There is nothing better!

Our ancestors loved wine fermented from grapes. Today's science has confirmed the health benefits of wine, many of which are derived from the seeds themselves. Concentrating those life-giving and even life-extending benefits into grape seed extract makes French grape seed extract (FGSE) a potent tool that should be part of every household's medicine cabinet. That's true whether you are suffering from one of the many diseases of aging or if, like all of us, you want to avoid them altogether.

A major part of FGSE's power comes from substances with the tongue-twisting name, oligomeric proanthocyanidins (OPCs).

Although OPCs are found in many plants, they are concentrated to extraordinary levels in grape seeds, hence their healing power. OPCs are probably the most potent antioxidants known to science.

What is an antioxidant? Cut an apple, and within a few minutes, it will begin to turn brown due to its exposure to oxygen. We call this "rusting." Squeeze a wedge of lemon on that apple right after you cut it, and it won't turn brown. The lemon is an antioxidant—it neutralizes the rusting caused by oxygen exposure.

Bear with us now.

While we need to breathe oxygen to stay alive, oxygen in our cells works just as destructively as it does on that plain apple. Your lifestyle choices and exposure to environmental toxins over a lifetime cause "rust" (actually the correct terminology is free radical oxygen molecules) that accumulate in your cells. That free radical oxygen exposure triggers chronic inflammation, opening the door to cell aging and genetic deterioration, and the diseases of aging, including cancer, heart disease, diabetes, Alzheimer's disease, and more.

At least 90% of all of our modern-day diseases are caused by oxidative stress and inflammation.

Wouldn't it be great if we could just squeeze lemon juice into every cell of our bodies? But seriously, there is something else we can do.

The Great Neutralizer

Lab studies show that OPCs are much more effective than **vitamin C** and **vitamin E** and virtually any type of food in neutralizing those destructive free radical oxygen molecules.

The antioxidant levels in French grape seed extract are so high they are quite literally off the scale. The ORAC (oxygen radical absorbance capacity) value of FGSE is so high it is difficult to accurately measure —even with modern equipment. ORAC values are a measure of the free-radical fighting capabilities of a particular food.

We know that French grape seed extract has an ORAC value of at least 20,000 per gram, higher than any other food! Compare this to blueberry, which has a rating of 96, dark chocolate powder at 56, and strawberries at 43 per gram.

Foods with high antioxidant power, like French grape seed extract, balance immune system responses to reduce long-term (chronic) inflammation and short-term (acute) inflammation that governs wound healing and allergic responses. This has profound effects on virtually every chronic disease known to science.

ORAC Values (per 1 gram)

French grape seed extract	20,000 or more
Ginger root	148
Elderberries	147
Cinnamon	131
Acai berries	102
Artichoke	94
Blueberries (raw)	96
Cranberries	90
Basil (dried)	61
Blackberries	59
Red wine (cabernet)	45
Sage (fresh)	32

—*Source US Department of Agriculture 2010*

Of course, we are talking about the *right* grape seed extract. There have been some cheap products on the market in recent years that have little or no value. So called grape seed extract from China can cost as little as $20 per kilo. In this case, you get what you pay for.

The best quality grape seed extract comes from tannin-free French OPC grapes that have a small molecular structure for the best absorbability—and the raw materials cost twenty times as much. It's truly worth it, as you'll see as you progress through this book.

Combatting Cancer

The coming chapters will give you many more details on cutting edge new research that has catapulted this unique herbal formulation to the forefront of natural approaches to cancer.

We know that some natural substances—like FGSE and the OPCs within—can repair genetic damage and tell cancer-preventive genes to wake up and do their job. They can also signal overactive genes to calm down and behave in a normal manner rather than reproducing wildly. We know OPCs can eliminate cancer stem cells, the main reason why even "successful" cancer treatment almost always ends with a recurrence.

Here's a sneak preview of the extensive number of ways that FGSE and its OPCs target cancer. It is scientifically proven to:

- Reduce tumor size
- Stop cells from becoming cancerous
- Relieve inflammation, an underlying cause of cancer
- Stop the formation of blood vessels that feed cancerous tumors (angiogenesis)
- Signal cancerous cells to commit suicide (apoptosis)
- Target cancer stem cells, the primary reason why cancers spread (metastasis)

- Awaken sleeping genes that stop cancerous cell's growth or slow down genes that are telling cells to reproduce wildly (epigenetics)
- Protect smokers
- Overcome the body's natural rejection of chemotherapy drugs over time (chemoresistance)
- Work synergistically with other natural treatments, including curcumin
- Enhance conventional chemotherapy treatments while protecting healthy cells and organs (chemoprotection)

The first section of this book is primarily based on Dr. Goel's research on French grape seed extract and cancer. Still, it is impossible to separate the underlying causes of cancer from the causes of other diseases, especially inflammation and epigenetics (genes that do not reproduce exactly due to environmental, not inherited factors).

Most of his research has focused on colorectal cancer, one of the most common and deadly cancers in the U.S. and many Western countries.

Read on and learn all about the impressive anti-cancer properties of FGSE without the negative side effects of conventional cancer treatments and its power against other diseases of aging.

What You Need to Know

1. French grape seed extract is one of the most potent disease-fighting nutrients known to science.
2. The healing power of French grape seed extract is largely the result of its antioxidant and anti-inflammatory effects.
3. Science has proven that FGSE:
   - reduces inflammation
   - kills cancer cells and prevents their return
4. And grape seed extract (GSE):
   - prevents and reverses heart disease
   - improves blood sugar metabolism and blood sugar control in people with diabetes
   - protects brain cells from the plaque associated with Alzheimer's disease
   - speeds wound healing
   - wipes out 10 disease-causing bacteria, including the deadly MRSA
   - increases lifespan in lab animals

CHAPTER 2
A Powerful Natural Answer to Cancer

Cancer is one word that probably strikes more fear in the human heart than practically any other.

As well it should.

Even though more people are surviving cancer these days, the overall incidence of cancer is growing worldwide. While 18 million people were diagnosed with cancer globally in 2018, this number is expected to grow to 27.5 million new cancer cases by 2040.

As we approach the 50th anniversary of the 1971 U.S. War on Cancer, it's time to acknowledge that we are losing that war.

Yes, we have made some headway:

- Lung cancer deaths are down, mainly because fewer people are smoking, one of the primary causes of lung cancer. The number of smokers in the United States decreased by about one-third between 2005 and 2018.

- Colorectal cancer deaths have also declined, largely because more people undergo screening colonoscopies, which can help detect and eliminate polyps and small cancers before they become deadly.
- Breast cancer deaths decreased by about 34% from 1975-2006, but researchers theorize that the decrease is due to overdiagnosis in the 20th century rather than improved diagnostic or treatment techniques.

One in five men and one in six women worldwide will develop cancer during their lifetimes, and one in eight men and one in 11 women will die from the disease. Worldwide, the total number of people who are alive today— five years after a cancer diagnosis called the five-year prevalence— is estimated to be 43.8 million.

More than $100 billion has been spent on cancer research in the U.S. alone, resulting in a host of outrageously expensive and largely ineffective new drugs and the implementation of cutting-edge diagnostic techniques. Despite this enormous expenditure, the cancer death rate, adjusted for the population's size and age, has only decreased by 5% since 1950.

Those numbers are expected to increase dramatically in the coming years. The number of cancer cases in the U.S. is forecast to increase by 72% by 2035, and the number of cancer deaths will rise by 59% in the same time frame.

An even more sobering statistic: Worldwide, 9.6 million people died of cancer in 2018 alone. Those cancer victims are not just numbers. They are husbands and wives, mothers, fathers, brothers, sisters, best friends forever since elementary school, your next-door neighbor, and your colleagues at work.

If you have cancer, if you know anyone with cancer or if anyone you love has died of cancer, you might be feeling angry right now. Your anger would be well justified.

Why are we Losing the War on Cancer?

Here's the simple answer: We're losing the war on cancer because conventional medicine refuses to understand that each person's cancer is a unique and individual disease. There is no one-size-fits-all solution. Cancer is a terribly complex disease.

The newer and modern laser-targeted approaches to cancer treatment (a/k/a targeted therapy) will inevitably fail because cancer cells are smart— so smart they almost seem to have a brain. As soon as we target cancer cells from one direction, they change course and become resistant to whatever therapy worked last week or last month.

To successfully treat cancer, we must first understand the individual nature of each person's cancer. Then we must approach that cancer from a wide variety of ways. We need to *see* what will work this week and *anticipate* what will work next week because what will work in the future course of an individual's disease will assuredly be different than what has worked in the past.

Failure of the War on Cancer

Let's take a moment to go back and look at the War on Cancer. Our net gain against cancer in nearly 70 years is a paltry 5%.

We've made great strides against many other diseases.

Since 1950, we've cut heart disease deaths by more than 60%. We've slashed the number of deaths from strokes by two-thirds, and deaths from pneumonia and influenza are less than half what they were at mid-20th century. Yet our progress against cancer has been minimal.

Extrapolate the millions upon millions of cancer deaths since 1950, and it's easy to understand why every doctor, medical researcher, cancer patient, and cancer patient's family has every right to feel angry and frustrated.

President Richard Nixon declared war on cancer in his 1971 State of the Union address, vowing to "conquer this dread disease (and make the United States) . . . become the healthiest nation in the world."

Between 2008 and 2019, an average of 34 anti-cancer drugs have been approved or given fast track approval status by the FDA *every year*. FDA, increasing the feeding frenzy for the market against a wide range of cancers, including breast, colorectal, multiple myeloma, and prostate. Some of these drugs cost as much as $300,000 for one year's treatment, not to speak of surgeries, transplants, and associated expenses that can bankrupt a family.

All for nothing.

Yes, there are indeed cases where lives are saved or significantly prolonged with treatment, but at the same time, when you consider the numbers as a whole, we are making very little progress.

The best that cancer patients and their families could hope for with some of these "exciting" new drugs is at best a handful of months or weeks of life for their loved ones while giving them little relief from their suffering.

Here's some information on just one: Erbitux™, a chemotherapy agent for metastatic colorectal cancer, small cell lung cancer, and other head and neck cancers. It costs $89,000 a year and can be expected to add only six (miserable) weeks to a colorectal cancer patient's life. The National Institutes of Health has proclaimed it "not a cost-effective treatment." Plus, it has the usual side effects for chemotherapy drugs (nausea, vomiting, hair loss, lack of energy) and can have fatal side effects if other chemo drugs or radiation are being used.

That's just one drug. Think of literally hundreds of others, and you'll see that we are wasting money and precious human life because we are completely on the wrong track when it comes to treating and curing cancer.

Every single one of these expensive chemotherapy drugs has only one single target or addresses a single cancer pathway.

Dr. Goel can say with confidence that chemotherapy kills faster than cancer because:

- It suppresses the immune system, disabling the body's ability to disarm cancer cells and remove them from the body leaving the patient vulnerable to other diseases;
- It kills healthy cells along with cancer cells;
- It kills the most rapidly dividing cells, but not all cancer cells are fast- growing;
- Chemotherapy drugs do not kill cancer cells.

He has been researching cancer for more than 20 years, and he can say unequivocally that cancer is a different disease in every single case. That presents a real challenge in figuring out the best treatments.

Yes, there are commonalities in cancers, but cancer involves a complex roadmap of genes and pathways that can take on exponential numbers of possibilities. Therefore, approaching it with only one tool is fruitless. We need to approach cancer knowing that those smart cancer cells can adapt to the ever-evolving disease in each cancer patient and make drug treatment ineffective at an impressive speed.

In a new field called precision medicine, we consider at least 13 factors that give us a deep profile of each patient to help doctors decide which treatment is likely to be the most effective:

- Tumor genome and epigenome

- Disease presentation
- Socioeconomic status
- Metabolic profile
- Reproductive and medical factors and side effects for cancer and other diseases
- Immune profile
- Microbiome
- Geography
- Lifestyle and environmental exposures
- Gender and age
- Family history
- Race/ethnicity

What is Cancer?

Cancer is defined as the uncontrolled growth of abnormal cells in the body. Old cells do not die and instead grow out of control, forming new, abnormal cells. These extra cells often form masses of tissue, called tumors, but some cancers, such as leukemia, do not form tumors.

Tumors form because cells ignore the body's normal signaling that it's time to stop growing or it's time to die —a natural process called apoptosis. Cell signaling pathways that avoid the normal controls can cause the formation and growth of cancer.

Over time, cancerous cells multiply and form other tumors. Cancer stem cells enter the bloodstream, migrating the disease to another place in the body, a process called metastasis.

Impaired genes are always the underlying cause of cancer, but that's not what you might think. Yes, there are hereditary cancers, but the vast majority of cancers (more than 95%, in my opinion) are caused by epigenetics—gene damage caused by environmental factors, including dietary choices, smoking, toxic exposures, etc. Almost all of these are preventable—more on that in the coming chapters.

We *have* learned some things about cancer since the War on Cancer began more than 40 years ago.

Here it is in a nutshell. Cancerous cells have the following in common:

- Activated oncogenes (genes that cause cancer)
- Inactive tumor suppressor genes
- Failed cell suicide (apoptosis)
- No limit to cell divisions
- Increased angiogenesis—formation of blood vessels that feed cancerous tumors
- Increased metastasis—the ability to spread cancer to other tissues

How Does French Grape Seed Extract Fit Into This Picture?

You've already heard us call French grape seed extract "Mother Nature's multi-tasker." That's because it has scientifically proven effectiveness against a broad spectrum of modern-day diseases, many of them the diseases of aging.

From Dr. Goel:

When it comes to cancer, I have to confess that my team's findings have surpassed our wildest expectations over the past three years.

Most importantly, using a technique never used before, our team was able to confirm that OPCs stop the mechanism that transforms non-cancerous cells and "normal" cancer cells into specialized and deadly cancer stem cells. These cancer stems cells promote tumor growth, and they can lie dormant in the bloodstream, sometimes for years, only to awaken some time later, perhaps in the same place or possibly spreading the cancer to another place in the body. These time bomb stem cells explain why people who have had cancer and have been pronounced "cancer-free" often find themselves with the disease again years later.

This research means that OPCs not only stop the growth of cancerous tumors, they can also stop cancers from spreading, and perhaps they can even prevent cancer altogether.

In addition to telling cancer cells to die when their time comes, the OPCs in French grape seed extract also help kill cancerous tumors by cutting off their blood supply (angiogenesis) and stop the spread of cancer (metastasis) through a wide variety of "pathways," targeting cancer from several directions as is necessary to beat the disease. They even enhance the effectiveness of chemotherapy drugs and radiation therapy commonly used in conventional cancer treatment and help reduce side effects and damage to healthy organs. These discoveries are immensely exciting and prove that low-cost, non-toxic, plant-derived cancer treatments can be extremely effective.

What You Need to Know

- Cancer diagnosis and death rates have not changed significantly in the past 40 years, despite earlier detection techniques. This means that more cancers are occurring, probably because of our lifestyle and environment.
- Your lifestyle, particularly your eating choices, are the most powerful predictors of your lifelong health, your risk of colon cancer, heart disease, Alzheimer's disease, and the other commonly recognized "diseases of aging."
- We can rather easily change our risk of cancer by controlling environmental factors and lifestyle choices.
- French grape seed extract has now been scientifically confirmed to fight cancer in a variety of powerful ways, making it one of our most potent botanical weapons against this disease.

CHAPTER 3
A Shotgun Approach to Cancer

You may remember that in the last chapter, we said that all cancers are unique. No two people will respond identically to the same cancer treatment. That is because we are all different. That's the concept of bio-individuality.

Plus, cancer is multi-faceted. That means that just one approach will rarely wipe out a particular type of cancer.

And cancer is ever-evolving. That means that a treatment that worked last month or even last week may no longer be effective today for no apparent reason.

In this chapter, we'll explain how the power of the OPCs in French grape seed extract have unique abilities to target and defeat cancer in several ways:

1. Prevents carcinogenesis: Stop cells from becoming cancerous at all.
2. Inhibits tumorigenesis: Stop cancer cells from clumping together and forming advanced cancerous tumors.

3. Promotes apoptosis: Tell wildly reproducing cancer cells to return to their normal life cycles.
4. Inhibits angiogenesis: Stop tumors from building a blood supply to nourish and sustain them.
5. Reduces chemoresistance: Make conventional chemotherapy drugs effective.
6. Inhibits metastasis: Stop cancer from spreading.

Prevents Carcinogenesis

Carcinogenesis is just a fancy term for the beginning of cancer. We are still not sure what causes normal cells to begin to reproduce wildly and become cancerous. This means cancer cells can begin to clump together and form tumors, like those found in breast, prostate, lung, and many other cancers. In some cases, like in leukemia, multiple myeloma, and other blood cancers, there are no tumors. The disease is carried in the bloodstream.

If those normal cells continue on the pre-programmed path of life in which they are born, do what they were designed to do, and die on schedule, there is no problem. When they somehow deviate from that path, cancer can begin. We don't know exactly how or why this happens, but we know that lifestyle choices are certainly an important factor. This is especially true with about 90% of colorectal cancer and dietary choices.

So, the ultimate cancer treatment is to prevent it altogether.

OPCs have now been scientifically confirmed to do precisely that.

A study from Dr. Goel's team published in 2018 in the journal *Carcinogenesis,* showed that OPCs halted communication in all six known cancer cell-forming pathways. In simple terms, this means that normal cell life cycles cannot be disrupted, so cancer cannot begin. In his mind, this is a good reason for almost everyone to take French grape seed extract on an ongoing basis.

Let us add here that all of Dr. Goel's research by his team was done on colorectal cancer. However, there is ample scientific evidence that his results will also apply to many, if not most, other types of cancer, including deadly breast, lung, pancreatic, liver, and prostate cancers.

Inhibits Tumorigenesis

Tumorigenesis is the clumping together of abnormal cells to form tumors. Some experts use the term interchangeably with carcinogenesis. Dr. Goel thinks of it as the next step in the formation of cancers. In the case of tumor-forming cancer cells, they are different when those rogue cells begin to clump together.

In the study published in *Carcinogenesis*, Dr. Goel's team showed that OPCs were able to lock down those deviant cells and stop them from clumping together. They were also able to stop those rogue cells from moving around into positions where they can form tumors.

Promotes Apoptosis

While we're on the subject of abnormal cell behavior, let's talk about apoptosis, the process of a natural cellular life cycle. Normal cells are born to perform their function and die on schedule. Some, like skin cells, live only a couple of weeks. Others, like fat cells, hang around for about eight years while heart muscle cells live about 40 years, and brain cells are believed to live as long as 200 years! That raises many fascinating questions for another time.

When cells go rogue and don't die when they should, we have a problem. That's when they become cancerous and form tumors. One of the ways of targeting cancer is to stop that wild cell division and persuade cancerous cells to quite literally commit suicide, returning to their natural life cycles and die as they were genetically programmed to do. Dr. Goel's research shows that process, called apoptosis, is triggered by OPCs in French grape seed extract.

Inhibits Angiogenesis

All living things require nourishment in some form. Plants require sunshine, air, and water. Animals (including humans) need food, water, air, and sleep.

Cancerous tumors require a blood supply to carry nourishment to the tumors and allow it to grow and thrive. These tumors can grow a network of blood vessels to feed them, a process called angiogenesis.

It seems like a simple thing: If you cut off that network of blood vessels, the tumor will die. It does. But it's not just a matter of cutting away blood vessels from a tumor and allowing it to wither away. Think about carcinogenesis, tumorigenesis, and apoptosis, as I've explained in the previous pages. Then think about all of these things happening at one time. What is needed is something that will hit everything at once.

We do have such a substance: Our research proves that French grape seed extract and the super medicinal OPCs it contains cut off those blood vessels while it is multi-tasking a slew of other anti-cancer activities.

There are no pharmaceuticals with these kinds of abilities, mainly because conventional anti-cancer drugs throw those gene-signaling pathways out of balance. They further disrupt homeostasis and require other drugs to try to bring the body back in balance, creating a vicious circle and a downward spiral.

But there is hope, and there is an answer!

There are two other botanicals known to have similar properties: curcumin and andrographis. Stay with us. We'll talk about those in a few chapters.

Reduces Chemoresistance

In all Dr. Goel's years of cancer research, he has seen almost every cancer patient develop some degree of resistance to chemotherapy drugs.

This means that chemotherapy drugs that were effective in the earlier phases of treatment almost always stop working over time. The tumors become resistant to the drug's intended effects, and cancer cells continue to grow unchecked.

These cancer cells can be fooled once if they've never been exposed to a chemo drug before. The drug may initially destroy 95% or more of the cancer cells. But the cells the chemo does not kill are the ones left to reproduce. The "smart" cancer cells become resistant to that drug. Regardless of what we throw at them, they figure out how to develop resistance one way or another.

Cancer stem cells are even stronger and more resistant to conventional therapies than "normal" cancer cells.

The patient has already undergone at least one course of chemotherapy, complete with myriad side effects that can include nausea, hair loss, weight loss, muscle wasting, extreme fatigue, organ damage and more — only to learn that the cancer is not in remission or it has returned.

In these cases, the only option most doctors can offer is another course of chemotherapy with a different drug, administered in the hope a different drug will trick the genius cancer cells into dying on schedule.

The vicious circle has been set. Some of the cancer cells will die, but, until now, there have always been survivalist cancer cells that will hide out in the physiological wilderness and come back again another day.

Doctors try another form of chemo. The patient weakens. Quality of life deteriorates to the point where it becomes intolerable for the patient. The outcome has been set almost from the beginning: The doctors eventually announce they can offer nothing else to overcome those cancer cells. The patient, in utter despair at the thought of more life-consuming drugs, loses hope.

It's a horrible story that too many of us have witnessed, if not experienced for ourselves. It's heartbreaking. And it doesn't have to be this way at all.

Dr. Goel's OPC research published in *Carcinogenesis* in 2019 provides the hope that so many cancer patients seek.

In the simplest terms, OPCs combined with conventional chemotherapy drugs overcame the chemoresistance and resulted in substantial reductions in tumor size.

This is primarily accomplished by knocking down a virtual firewall called ABC transporters that keep chemo from reaching the tumor and killing it. See? I told you those cancer cells were incredibly smart.

Hopefully, we are smarter, or we are becoming smarter.

Not only do OPCs from French grape seed extract break down that chemoresistant firewall, reducing tumor growth within mere *hours*, they also sensitizes the cancer cells to the impact of the chemo drugs, meaning the patient needs fewer drugs and experiences fewer side effects.

Even better, the OPCs protect healthy cells, further minimizing the side effects of chemo drugs.

Metastasis

We'll be talking more about metastasis –the spread of existing cancer—in the next chapter when we get into cancer stem cells and the powerful effects OPCs have on them.

But let us say here that not only do OPCs reduce tumor growth, but they have also been scientifically proven to stop the spread of cancer when used with conventional chemotherapy drugs.

Dr. Goel is a scientist, not at all given to hyperbole, but wow. Just Wow! These findings are changing the way doctors treat their patients, even those with late-stage cancers, changing their chances of survival and offering them a vastly improved quality of life.

What You Need to Know

The OPCs in French grape seed extract have unique abilities to target cancer in several ways:

- Prevent carcinogenesis: Stop cells from becoming cancerous at all.
- Inhibit tumorigenesis: Stop cancer cells from clumping together and forming cancerous tumors.
- Promote apoptosis: Tell wildly reproducing cancer cells to return to their normal life cycles.
- Inhibit angiogenesis: Stop tumors from building a blood supply to nourish and sustain them.
- Reduce chemoresistance: Make conventional chemotherapy drugs effective.
- Inhibit metastasis: Stop cancer from spreading.

CHAPTER 4
Wipe Out Cancer Stem Cells

We are sure that you know someone who has had cancer. You most likely also know someone who had cancer and had all the conventional treatments, which can include surgery, chemotherapy, and radiation. After that they were declared "cancer-free." Three or four years later, maybe even longer, the cancer returned. Perhaps it was in the same location or elsewhere on the body. Maybe you know someone for whom cancer has returned three or more times.

This is heartbreaking.

As we've said in the previous chapters, cancer is an extremely complex disease. Cancer often returns after a long and grueling cancer treatment because cancer cells are smart and can evolve into cancer stem cells.

Cancer cells are the geniuses of the biochemical world. They're undoubtedly smarter than your average brain or bone or skin cell. Cancer cells are driven for self-preservation, with strength far beyond the survival instincts of normal cells. Like all life forms, they fight like demons to survive, but they are also incredibly intelligent, intelligent enough to thwart most attempts to kill them. It's almost like they have their own brains.

Those resistant cancer cells find a way to hide and survive, and some eventually emerge again and thrive. These are cancer stem cells, and they can be deadly. When cancers return, they tend to be far more vicious and more aggressive than they were the first time around and far more resistant to cancer treatments.

When a child is conceived, the egg and the sperm divide into a handful of healthy stem cells. Stem cells are the point of origination for all tissues in the body. Malleable like a child's Play-Doh, stem cells can become any kind of cell. They can be brain cells, heart cells, pancreas cells, skin cells or hair and nail cells. Stem cells are the superheroes of the body, capable of unlimited potential.

Cancer stem cells are different. We are not born with cancer stem cells. They are a tiny subset of cancer cells themselves—so named because they can be the point of origination for a cancer recurrence. They can disguise themselves and lie low, avoiding chemo and radiation therapy. When the coast is clear, they can spring forward and start making cancer cells again.

Cancer stem cells initiate and maintain cancer and contribute to recurrence and drug resistance, which we'll explore in the next chapter.

Cancer stem cells have immortality – or near-immortality. Think of them as super-cells. As we've learned in earlier chapters, cancer cells do not have a normal lifespan like healthy cells. They live on and on, reproducing in their twisted fashion, creating more cancer cells and larger tumors that can spread throughout the body. They can also send messages to the cancer cells to resist chemotherapy drugs.

These cancer stem cells have an uncanny ability to hide from conventional medicine's diagnostic "radar," lurking in the body's deepest recesses, appearing to sleep or staying quiet for months, even years, before they awaken and begin to grow again with a vengeance.

Not only that, but some ordinary cancer cells can transform themselves into cancer stem cells, increasing their power exponentially.

You'll note we said, "most," but not "all" attempts to kill cancer stem cells have failed. Conventional medicine offers absolutely nothing that can touch them.

Understanding and eliminating cancer stem cells is the cutting edge of cancer research today.

But there is now enormous hope: The latest research has confirmed that a botanical treatment is astonishingly effective against the best-laid plans of cancer cells.

There is Hope

Dr. Goel was honored to lead a creative and brilliant research team at Baylor University. He headed the Center for Gastrointestinal Research and the Center for Epigenetics, Cancer Prevention, and Cancer Genomics in Dallas until the summer of 2019.

This team was the first to create organoids for research in botanical treatments for cancer. These are tiny three-dimensional versions of cancerous tumors. They then subjected the organoids to various substances without having to involve or harm a human patient. Think of those organoids as stand-ins identical to the actual tumors.

Organoids are conglomerations of cells, but the unique thing is that they are exact 3D replicas of the cancerous tumors in real human patients. In the past, we have been able to work with laboratory-generated cell lines and animals, but, for ethical reasons, it is extremely complicated to do research on human subjects. Now we can take an exact replica of human tumors outside the patient's body, look directly into them, and discover precisely what will work to kill them.

Remember, Dr. Goel said that each patient's cancer is individual and requires unique ways of treating it? These stand-in clones of the actual tumor give us a perfect way to discover the treatments that work as opposed to lab-grown cell cultures or animal experimentation, which may or may not reflect how a given substance might act in humans.

The immensely exciting discovery from our research team is this: French grape seed extract is enormously effective in killing cancer stem cells.

Let us repeat that: The OPCs in French grape seed extract *killed* cancer stem cells. Other than curcumin (stay with me for more on that), French grape seed extract is the *only* substance, natural or pharmaceutical in our experience that stops cancer stem cells from reproducing.

In Dr. Goel's lab, we exposed cancer organoids to OPCs and found that in just five days, the presence of cancer in those organoids was dramatically decreased.

These unique studies are the only ones done using human-derived organoids. It proves that botanicals like French grape seed extract can be used for precisely targeted cancer treatments.

Hippo Pathway

Remember those ordinary cancer cells that have somehow acquired a superpower to transform themselves into cancer stem cells?

The OPCs in French grape seed extract have that problem in hand, too.

All cells, including cancer cells, communicate with each other. Think of it as an electrical network. So, what happens if one part of that network is cut? The entire network fails.

With cancer, a network called Hippo (no need to go into the complex science behind this one!) is responsible for carrying the signal that tells those ordinary cancer cells to morph into cancer stem cells. But what if the Hippo network is interrupted? No new cancer stem cells form, *and* existing cancer stem cells can no longer reproduce. Cancer becomes much easier to treat and destroy.

While Dr. Goel's team's breakthrough research is on colorectal cancer, we are confident, and voluminous other research has confirmed, it will translate to a wide variety of other types of cancer.

This research now gives us the strongest possible evidence that French grape seed extract is an inexpensive, non-toxic way to stop the formation of cancer stem cells. The implications for these discoveries in future cancer treatment and prevention are very exciting.

What You Need to Know

- Cancer stem cells are insidious types of cancer cells that can carry cancer to other parts of the body long after a patient has been declared "cancer-free."
- Dr. Goel's research on test tube-like cancers actually extracted from patients with colorectal cancer shows that OPCs in French grape seed extract can eradicate cancer stem cells, preventing cancer from recurring or spreading in humans, not just in laboratory cell cultures or animal research.
- OPCs can stop ordinary cancer cells from morphing into cancer stem cells that have superpowers to lurk in the body and re-emerge months or even years later.
- These breakthrough discoveries have profound implications for cancer treatment.

CHAPTER 5
The One-Two Punch

We've talked at length here about OPCs and their impressive ways of suppressing, fighting and eradicating cancer employing several methods all at once.

If that is not enough, what if there was another natural treatment that enhanced the already impressive power of FGSE?

Then imagine we put those together and discovered that combined, their power against cancer was multiplied?

That's exactly what Dr. Goel's research team found: If you add the OPCs in French grape seed extract to the verified anti-cancer powers of curcumin, we have a one-two punch against cancer that can't be beat.

In their study published in *Scientific Reports* in 2018, his team found that the botanical combination was doubly effective in preventing carcinogenesis (failures in cell reproduction that start the cancer process) and enhanced other anti-cancer weapons.

The results were so important that they concluded: "We make a case for the clinical co-administration of curcumin and OPCs as a treatment therapy for patients with colorectal cancer."

From Dr. Goel: Let me add here that in my tenure as a cancer researcher, not only have I deeply studied French grape seed extract and OPCs, I have also engaged in years of research on curcumin and its impressive anti-cancer effects.

In my 2016 book, Curcumin: Nature's Answer to Cancer and Other Chronic Diseases, I stated the following unequivocally: "Curcumin is the only substance known to science that targets cancer from so many directions at once. I say this without qualification. Curcumin is a natural substance, and it is the only substance, natural or synthetic, that science has proven addresses and combats cancer in so many different ways."

Now I am proud to say that French grape seed extract OPCs join curcumin's elite status. Our research shows that hand-in-hand, the anti-cancer powers of these two botanicals exceeded our wildest expectations.

It's also important to remember that, although my research has been focused on botanicals and colorectal cancer, numerous studies have confirmed that those results apply in addition to many, if not most, other types of cancer.

In the first four chapters of this book, you've received a thorough explanation of how French grape seed extract OPCs can prevent, treat, and even eradicate colorectal cancer.

The Power of Curcumin

Now let's take a look at curcumin and its impressive effects.

If you love curry, you'll be familiar with turmeric, a popular, vividly colored golden spice.

Turmeric in itself has a plethora of health benefits, if, like people in India, you're willing to eat it in huge quantities several times a day beginning in childhood. Botanically known as *Curcuma longa*, the turmeric rhizome is a member of the antioxidant-rich ginger family.

Inside turmeric is a compound called curcumin, which is found in its rhizome (the stem of the plant found underground). However, there is very little curcumin in the spice turmeric. If you've seen cheap turmeric supplements on the market, understand that they only contain 2% to 5% curcumin, which may or may not be usable by your body. They're not likely to have much effectiveness in preventing or treating the diseases we're talking about. Curcumin is *many times* more powerful than turmeric.

In simple terms, turmeric is the spice and curcumin is the medicine.

Curcumin has shown positive effects in treating every single disease for which it has been studied.

For years, we have thought curcumin's anti-inflammatory, antioxidant, and anti-cancer properties were unique in the plant world. Now we know that French grape seed extract and its OPCs have similar properties that act with curcumin to compound their healing properties.

The One-Two Punch

Remember from Chapter 3, how OPCs fight cancer?

- carcinogenesis (the formation of cancerous cells)
- tumorigenesis (the formation of tumors)
- apoptosis (cells that refuse to die at the end of their natural lives, creating cancers)
- angiogenesis (the formation of a blood supply to feed and nourish cancerous tumors)
- chemoresistance (failure of conventional chemotherapy drugs over time)
- metastasis (the spread of cancer to other parts of the body)
- cancer stem cells that hide from treatment, allowing the disease to go dormant and then appear months or years later

Duplicate this list for curcumin. It does all of the above. Curcumin checks all the cancer-fighting boxes.

Have you heard of the term "synergy?"

The Oxford dictionary defines it as "the interaction or cooperation of two or more organizations, substances, or other agents to produce a combined effect greater than the sum of their separate effects."

We don't understand why, but we have confirmed that the two botanicals together have vastly more healing power than either has individually. We call it the One-Two Punch.

Even at lower dosages, the natural combination was more effective than treatment with either OPCs or curcumin alone. This was especially true when the One-Two Punch was aimed at cells that had become resistant to conventional chemotherapy drugs.

Using organoids (remember those tiny, lab-grown, exact duplicates of human patients' tumors?), Dr. Goel's study showed the two were highly effective at stopping cancer cells from forming, at stopping apoptosis and at boosting the effects of conventional chemotherapy, even when patients were given half doses of each.

The One-Two Punch targets cancer in several ways, each perhaps only infinitesimally different from the other, covering even more bases than either one individually.

It does all of this without damaging any healthy cells and without side effects.

What that means is that when you add super bioavailable curcumin to OPCs from French grape seed extract you get a healing combination that has the potential to relegate cancer to the annals of medical history.

A Bonus!

The latest research suggests there is another powerhouse combo and overcomes chemoresistance: FGSEs and *andrographis paniculata*, an herb used in Ayurvedic medicine.

Most people (85-90%) with advanced colorectal cancers do not respond to commonly used chemotherapy drugs. Doctors must often switch chemo drugs to get any positive results until multi-drug resistance is almost inevitable, and doctors run out of options.

We already know that combination therapies are the most effective. Dr. Goel's team is working on identifying how FGSE and andrographis can team up to fight colorectal cancers and other difficult-to-treat cancers.

Stay tuned!

What You Need to Know

- We already know that the OPCs in French grape seed extract are powerful fighters against cancer from a variety of directions.
- Past research confirms that bioavailable curcumin has many of the same capabilities against cancer.
- New research shows that combining OPCs from French grape seed extract and curcumin works synergistically—more potently than either individually—to fight cancer in a variety of ways.
- The combination is safe and very effective against cancers that have stopped responding to conventional chemotherapy.
- It can restore the effectiveness of conventional chemotherapy drugs at lower dosages and minimizes side effects.

PART 2:
French Grape Seed Extract's Power Against Other Diseases

CHAPTER 6
Insidious Inflammation and Obdurate Oxidation

Inflammation and oxidation are underlying causes of virtually every disease of aging. Stop those fires of inflammation and oxidation, and you have slowed down the disease process of aging. It's that simple.

The Inflammatory Cascade

Let's start with inflammation.

There are two basic types of inflammation: acute inflammation and chronic inflammation. If you've ever sprained an ankle, whacked your thumb with a hammer, or been stung by a bee—the swelling, redness, and heat you noticed are all part of the healing process. You experienced acute inflammation, an important component of the recovery process associated with an injury.

Here's how it works: When you get a tissue injury, your body's immune system sends out white blood cells to neutralize the inflammation. This is the human body's natural response to an injury. Your sprained ankle, bee sting, or whacked thumb will hurt for a while, maybe requiring a little pain medicine or ice, and then it heals on its own, thanks to white blood cells and the innate healing power of the human body.

However, there's another type of inflammation that is far more insidious. Chronic inflammation may begin as acute inflammation but does not resolve for a number of reasons. This is the type of inflammation that can be associated with longstanding pain, as in the case of osteoarthritis.

Yet another type of chronic inflammation is far more subtle. It usually has no outward signs of pain or no symptoms at all. It may go completely unnoticed, as in the case of obesity, cardiovascular disease, diabetes, cancer, and neurodegenerative diseases like Alzheimer's disease. Whether or not there is pain, these diseases and others are the direct result of inflammation.

Chronic inflammation is the spark that ignites disease. When chronic inflammation continues unchecked, it disrupts biological functions, damaging healthy cells and triggering inappropriate immune responses, eventually leading to DNA damage, tissue death, and internal scarring.

Chronic inflammation is almost always caused by lifestyle choices and by environmental factors including:

- eating processed and adulterated foods, especially sugar, excessive refined carbohydrates, and vegetable oils

- overeating
- smoking
- breathing polluted air
- drinking municipal water
- using toxic personal care products (shampoo, soap, toothpaste, makeup, deodorant, and more)
- toxic cleaning products
- petrochemicals and gas fumes
- pesticides and herbicides
- living and working in toxic environments (off-gassing carpets, furniture, and bedding)

The Big S

Let's add in what may be the major cause of chronic inflammation: The Big S: STRESS. Long-term unrelieved stress, like most of us experience every single day, interferes with the ability of the stress hormone, cortisol, to stimulate the immune system and control inflammation, according to a 2012 study from Carnegie Mellon University. Researchers found that highly stressed people were substantially more likely to get colds when exposed to the cold virus as opposed to people whose lower stress levels promoted healthy immune function.

Beyond the higher risk of viral infections, unrelenting stress clearly opens the door to all of those diseases we want to avoid.

We'll say this in the simplest terms possible: If you are obese or have diabetes, heart disease, Alzheimer's disease, or cancer, you have a disease triggered by chronic inflammation. These are lifestyle diseases. While you may not be able to control the air pollution in your town or the off-gassing furniture and carpet in your office, there are healthy lifestyle choices you can make that will minimize your risk of chronic inflammation and the inflammatory diseases we all want to avoid.

If you don't have these diseases yet, paying attention to the lifestyle choices you can control and managing stress will go a long way toward protecting you.

And, of course, you can take French grape seed extract. While nothing will 100% guarantee that you never become obese or get heart disease, cancer, diabetes, or Alzheimer's disease, FGSE is one of the best life insurance policies the herbal world offers.

Oxidation

Oxygen is the key to life. If we are deprived of oxygen for even a few minutes, the consequences are grave, even fatal. So, what is oxygen doing that makes it so critically important?

Oxygen is the substance solely utilized by the 1,500 or so mitochondria found in every cell of our bodies. These are the energy-producing bodies that create the necessary electricity (energy) that allows us to function. Those mitochondria are like hydroelectric power plants. The oxygen that flows through the mitochondria is like the water that falls down the dams and turns the turbines, creating energy. Imagine if we didn't have this energy production, we wouldn't be able to function!

On the other hand, oxygen is a double-edged sword. Not only does it create the energy (electricity) needed for life, but it also produces oxidation.

We gave the examples of an oxidizing apple in an earlier chapter. The browning of a cut apple slice (rusting) is caused by the cells on the apple's surface reacting with oxygen.

Think about rust on the bumper of your car. Scientifically, this "rust" is caused by unstable oxygen molecules missing an electron or two. Unstable oxygen molecules, called free radicals, cause "rust" on your cells, damaging DNA in much the same way they cause an apple to brown. It also causes cellular reproduction to be disrupted, so new cells are not exact copies of the parent cells. This is how aging cells open the way to diseases, especially unnatural cell growth.

Our bodies are bombarded by free radical oxygen molecules 24/7. Toxins in air, food, water, cigarette smoke, industrial pollutants, pesticides, herbicides, and other environmental toxins contribute to the free radical population explosion.

Yet, we are not helpless against this onslaught. Antioxidants found in plants, foods, and nutrients, neutralize free radicals and can even donate electrons to help stabilize these electrically challenged oxygen molecules and neutralize their destructive potential.

Antioxidants like those found in grape seed extract are among the most powerful forces we have against free radical damage and disease.

Oxidative stress is the body's ability to combat those free radical oxygen molecules with antioxidant defense to keep the body healthy and balanced.

Andrew Weil, M.D., one of our favorite holistic physicians, says, "Health depends on a balance between oxidative stress and antioxidant defenses. Aging and age-related diseases reflect the inability of our antioxidant defenses to cope with oxidative stress over time. The good news is that with strong antioxidant defenses, long life without disease should be possible."

Quenching the Fires of Inflammation and Oxidation

The best news is that we have control over both inflammation and oxidation.

FGSE has hundreds of potent healing properties, but probably none are as important or as basic to human health as its ability to fight inflammation and oxidation.

Inflammation

It works as an anti-inflammatory in much the same way as NSAIDs (non-steroidal anti-inflammatory drugs like aspirin, ibuprofen, naproxen, and prescription drugs like Voltaren, Bextra, and Celebrex) without the serious side effects that have been connected to these drugs.

NSAIDs are used to relieve pain related to inflammation, including arthritis pain. They also inhibit the COX-2 enzyme, which can lead to serious and sometimes fatal gastrointestinal problems and increase the risk of heart attacks and strokes.

FGSE has all of the anti-inflammatory benefits of NSAIDS and no negative side effects.

Research shows that OPCs prevent the body from manufacturing prostaglandins, the major inflammatory hormone that triggers inflammation as well as causing blood clot formation, the constriction of blood vessels. They also regulate the contraction and relaxation of the muscles in the digestive system and airways.

Oxidation

OPCs are highly effective free radical scavengers, interrupting the chain reaction of disease-causing cellular deterioration and repairs radical damage.

OPCs are formidable warriors against disease themselves with their stratospheric ORAC scores, as mentioned in Chapter 1.

In addition to their own antioxidant power, OPCs can actually jump-start the antioxidant, anti-clotting, anti-inflammatory, and anti-tumor properties of the already formidable effects of vitamins C and E.

They also stop the formation of Nuclear Factor kappa B (better known as NF-kB), one of the most powerful markers of inflammation that also controls cell survival and the programmed cell death that is necessary to keep the cells from dividing wildly and causing cancers and other disease and the duplication of DNA in cells (when that goes wonky, the cells reproduce imperfectly, causing a wide range of problems, including cancer).

The best grape seed OPC extract is one that can show the highest possible ORAC value. ORAC values are a way of determining how much free radical fighting power a given fruit or vegetable has. While there's no way of duplicating the complex structure and synergy of a food, there are improved ways of taking some of the best components of fruits and vegetables and concentrating them to the point where you see extremely high ORAC values. One studied extract has an ORAC value of over 21,000 per gram!

What You Need to Know

- Chronic inflammation and oxidation (free radical damage) are silent killers that are the underlying cause of virtually all of the diseases of aging: heart disease, diabetes, cancer, and Alzheimer's disease.
- Since there are often no identifiable symptoms of chronic inflammation and oxidative damage, there is no way to know you have that without medical testing— or until you develop one of the diseases they cause.
- Stress is a major cause of inflammation.
- Lifestyle choices, including what you eat, your exercise regimen, and your exposure to environmental toxins, can cause chronic inflammation and free radical damage to your cells.
- OPCs like those found in French grape seed extract are among the most powerful warriors known to science to combat inflammation and oxidation.

CHAPTER 7
A Guardian Against Heart Disease

French grape seed extract is no doubt your heart's best friend. Of all the considerable powers of this tiny seed, heart disease prevention and control is arguably one of its greatest strengths.

A study published in the medical journal *Lancet* in 1993 is foundational to today's knowledge of how OPCs protect the heart. Of 805 men studied by Dutch researchers, those who consumed the most flavonoids (compounds like those found in many fruits and vegetables and especially in grape seed extract) had the lowest risk of a heart attack. Conversely, those with the lowest flavonol intake had a very high risk of heart attack and an even greater risk of death from a heart attack.

Heart disease is the #1 killer in the world, for both men and women. The numbers are a bit daunting. They should be more than a little bit scary, and they should get your attention:

- Cardiovascular disease (heart attacks, strokes, and other cardiovascular disease) killed 17.9 million people worldwide, accounting for approximately 31% of all deaths from all causes.
- By 2030, that number is expected to increase by more than one-third to 23.6 million.
- Although most of us think of heart disease as the product of a relatively opulent Western lifestyle, 85% of cardiovascular disease deaths take place in low- and middle-income countries.
- It claims more lives than all types of cancers combined.
- Nearly half of all African-American adults have some form of cardiovascular disease.

—*Source: American Heart Association and World Health Organization*

So, should we be afraid of heart disease? You bet we should, for all the grim reasons cited above.

Is there anything you can do to prevent this onward march of death?

Absolutely!

Lifestyle choices are probably the greatest strategy for heart disease prevention.

Here are the simple ones that you probably already know, but you hope they don't apply to you:

The Super 7 Strategies to Prevent Heart Disease

1. Don't smoke!
2. Get moving! Exercise at least 30 minutes every day.
3. Eat less sugar, more fruits, veggies, whole grains, and healthy fats.
4. Control your weight.
5. Control your blood pressure.
6. Control your cholesterol.
   a. Don't worry so much about lowering your cholesterol, be more concerned about lowering your triglycerides (blood fats) and increasing your HDL cholesterol.
   b. Note— it's oxidized LDL cholesterol that is a contributing factor to heart disease (there is oxidation appearing yet again).
7. Control your blood sugar.

Now, we know that many of our readers have already heard all of the strategies above. You probably also know that #3 —a healthy diet—has a heavy influence on four of the others: controlling weight, cholesterol, blood pressure, and blood sugar.

We won't reiterate all of the sermons you've heard from your doctors or read in the press, but we can tell you there is a lot of truth here. It is worth your life to pay attention.

And adding high-quality French grape seed extract to your daily supplement regimen is a wise choice, too. Think of it as an insurance policy for the healthy choices you are already making.

Here's why: Numerous solid scientific studies show that grape seed extract covers four of the Super 7 strategies *plus* it helps prevent diabetes, a major risk for heart disease. We'll talk about that in the next chapter.

Lowers Blood Pressure

Probably the most exciting study of grape seed extract and blood pressure came from Italy, where 119 people with pre- or mild hypertension were given either 150 mg or 300 mg of grape seed extract a day. A control group was given diet and lifestyle recommendations with no assistance from any supplements or medications. The results showed both grape seed groups reduced their blood pressure substantially, but surprisingly, the lower dosage was more effective in reducing blood pressure than the higher dosage. In four months, blood pressure returned to normal in an impressive 93% of the lower dose group.

A similar study from the Illinois Institute for Technology confirmed the Italian study's results and found that grape seed extract lowered systolic blood pressure (the upper number) by 5-6% and diastolic (the lower number) by 4-7% with no negative side effects. As a bonus, they found the grape seed extract group had lower fasting insulin and improved insulin sensitivity, something important for people with diabetes who are also at high risk for heart disease.

An animal study from the University of Alabama at Birmingham attempted to mimic the increased risk for high blood pressure in women after menopause. In a University of Nevada study, rats fed a poor diet had lower blood pressure, the grape seed extract even seemed to neutralize the hypertensive effects of a high salt diet. In addition, the grape seed extract seemed to enhance the animals' ability to neutralize those dangerous free radical oxygen molecules.

Strengthens and Relaxes Blood Vessel Walls

There is evidence that grape seed extract allows blood vessel walls to relax, allowing blood to flow freely through them with less force, further reducing blood pressure. It also helps activate an important enzyme called nitric oxide synthase, producing nitric oxide that relaxes blood vessel walls as well as regulating the production of the dangerous inflammatory protein NF-kB that can make blood vessels more rigid.

It also increases collagen production, the protein that connects muscles, bones, tendons, and, yes, blood vessels. Why is this important? Think of a fire hose. If it's strong, it can withstand the intense pressure of the water that passes through it. Strong blood vessel walls are better able to withstand high blood flow and even high blood pressure without rupturing, as happens in certain types of strokes.

In simple terms, the OPCs in grape seed extract strengthens blood vessels while making them more flexible.

Reduces Cholesterol and Triglycerides

French grape seed extract turns out to be a formidable opponent of arterial plaque and elevated blood fats.

Excess cholesterol and elevated triglycerides can combine with fat, excess calcium, and other substances in the blood to cause inflammation and eventually forming plaque. These fatty deposits in the blood vessels can subsequently clog arteries; a disease called atherosclerosis, literally hardening of the arteries. Some blocked arteries may rupture in time, causing a heart attack or stroke.

The oxidation of LDL (low density lipoprotein) cholesterol, the type considered the most dangerous by most doctors, is one of the first steps on the road to a heart attack.

Stay with us a moment—this gets a bit complicated:

A significant study from Georgetown University concluded that patients with high cholesterol (between 200 and 300 mg/dL) who took grape seed extract reduced autoantibodies to oxidized LDL cholesterol by an impressive 50%. Oxidized LDL cholesterol is a particularly dangerous type of blood fat that has reacted with those free radical oxygen molecules we have talked about in previous chapters. When LDL cholesterol is oxidized, it produces long-term inflammation and tissue damage, and, in the case of heart disease, increases risks of heart attack and stroke dramatically.

So, this Georgetown study is important to anyone with elevated cholesterol and even more important to people who already have been diagnosed with heart disease and/or diabetes precisely because of its potent antioxidant properties to help neutralize this type of cholesterol.

A Spanish animal study confirmed the value of grape seed extract in treating high cholesterol. It normalized cholesterol in rats and even protected against fatty liver, an excess cholesterol condition related to obesity, among other things.

An impressive animal study from the University of Nevada at Reno showed how effective grape seed extract is at reversing the effects of high triglycerides (fats in the bloodstream) that greatly increase the risk of heart disease. When researchers gave laboratory animals a super high fructose diet for eight weeks, all their triglyceride numbers shot up a frightening 171%! But animals given the same diet plus grape seed extract *reduced* their triglycerides by 41%.

Before we get too far with this line of thinking, we want to note that grape seed extract is not a magic bullet. Taking French grape seed extract does not mean you can eat a terrible diet and neutralize all of the negative effects by taking this powerful supplement.

Reduces the Risk of Blood Clots

In addition to the risks posed by narrowed arteries, blood clots contribute to the risk of cardiovascular disease. The two combined can be lethal.

Grape seed OPCs prevent blood clots, thus offering powerful protection against heart attacks and strokes.

Grape seed extract reduces blood levels of fibrinogen, the clotting factor, preventing clots from forming and dissolving clots that may already exist.

It can directly bust clots before they can form, according to a 2005 Japanese lab and animal study. A Polish study published in 2012 cited grape seed extract's ability to protect against clotting as part of its considerable antioxidant properties.

What You Need to Know

- Heart disease is the #1 cause of death worldwide.
- Grape seed extract's impressive antioxidant and anti-inflammatory effects protect against heart disease by:
    o Lowering blood pressure
    o Strengthening blood vessel walls while making them more flexible
    o Lowering LDL cholesterol
    o Lowering triglycerides
    o Reducing the risk of blood clots that cause heart attacks and strokes

CHAPTER 8
A Tool in the Fight Against Metabolic Syndrome, Type 2 Diabetes, and Obesity

Metabolic syndrome, obesity, and diabetes are an intertwined basket of health issues that add up to serious, and even life-threatening, consequences.

Our modern lifestyle has mired us in these diseases. Much of our collective problems are directly linked to the Standard American Diet (SAD) of high sugar and highly processed foods, a sedentary lifestyle, and unrelieved stress.

Read on to understand more and to learn how French grape seed extract can help you overcome these dastardly health risks.

Metabolic Syndrome

Let's start with metabolic syndrome. This is a collection of symptoms – or health markers – that can cause heart disease, stroke, and diabetes, if they are not addressed.

There are five conditions that the medical profession generally agrees comprise metabolic syndrome:

- **Large waistline:** Belly fat is dangerous, pure, and simple. An apple-shaped figure and/or that dreaded beer belly are sure signs that you are at risk.
- **High triglyceride levels:** If your blood work shows your triglycerides over 150 mg/dL, or if you are on triglyceride-lowering prescription drugs, you are at risk. What this means is those excess carbohydrate calories you consume are stored in your fat cells. There is some evidence that high triglyceride levels contribute to atherosclerosis— hardening of the arteries —and, at extremely high levels, to acute pancreatitis.
- **Low levels of HDL cholesterol:** HDL or the so-called "good" cholesterol is what you need to balance the effects of LDL cholesterol, which can increase the risk of heart disease. So, in the case of cholesterol, the higher the HDL number, the better. In men, this is at least 40 mg/dL and women, 50 mg/dL.
- **High blood pressure:** Elevated pressure of blood rushing through arteries can, over time, lead to plaque buildup as coronary artery disease, if your blood pressure is consistently over the ideal reading of 120/80 mm Hg. Medical science has recently

adjusted those numbers to keep a "normal" reading of 140/90 mm Hg, although it's safer to keep your numbers in that lower range.
- **High fasting blood sugar:** Even mildly high blood sugar can be a sign of early diabetes. When you awaken in the morning before you eat or drink anything, normal blood sugar should be between 70 and 100 mg/dL. Anything from 101-126 mg/dL signals impaired glucose tolerance, and anything above 126 mm/dL is diagnostic of diabetes. If you know someone who has a blood sugar monitor, it's easy to do a nearly painless finger stick blood test. If not, your doctor's office can do it, or have it done at any number of clinics.

If you have three or more of these risk factors, you have metabolic syndrome. The more of these risk factors you have, the greater your risk for heart disease, stroke, or diabetes.

The *Journal of the American Medical Association* reported in 2015 that nearly 35% of the American adult population and 50% of the population over the age of 60 have metabolic syndrome.

Obesity

Please read over the list of metabolic syndrome risk factors above. All of them are directly associated with obesity. As a nation, we are becoming fatter and fatter. And it turns out; it's not just a national problem. It's global.

Nearly four in ten (39.6%) of American adults are obese, according to the Centers for Disease Control and Prevention (CDC). It's even more alarming that this figure is almost *triple* for the worldwide obesity levels. Another startling fact? Nearly three-quarters of American men and 60% of American women are overweight or obese. Statistic show that 30% of our children are obese.

Obesity is a disease. Not only does obesity increase the risk for metabolic syndrome, according to the National Heart Lung and Blood Institute, it also vastly increases the risk of heart disease, stroke, and diabetes. Sound familiar?

Obesity also increases the risk of cancer, especially colon and breast cancer, along with osteoarthritis, sleep apnea, infertility, and fatty liver disease.

The underlying causes of obesity and the ways to fight it could be the subject of several books, but let us say that a healthy diet and active lifestyle could quite literally save your life.

Inflammation is part of the link here, which will become clearer when we start talking about grape seed extract in a few pages. Inflammation, the silent killer, is a huge cause of chronic diseases, including obesity.

Exciting new research just published in the Journal of Ethnopharmacology shows that grape seed OPCs have another superpower rare in the plant world: they can cross the blood-brain barrier and suppress leptin, the appetite-stimulating hormone that contributes to overeating and obesity.

French grape seed extract supplementation gives you one of the most formidable tools science has against obesity, a disease that is extremely difficult to treat and reverse.

Diabetes

Type 2 diabetes was once called "adult onset diabetes" and was mostly the domain of people over 50. In recent years, that signature has been dropped because we've experienced an epidemic of obesity in children and teenagers. The result has been a similar alarming rise in type 2 diabetes among young people. More than 90% of people with this form of diabetes are overweight.

The increasing prevalence of type 2 diabetes has closely paralleled the obesity epidemic, with nearly 10% of the adult population (30.2 million people in 2012) with the disease. However, 28% of them do not know they have it, according to the CDC. Another 84 million or more have elevated blood sugar and are at high risk for developing type 2 diabetes in the next five years. Worse yet, CDC researchers project that 40% of Americans currently alive will develop type 2 diabetes in their lifetimes.

Type 2 diabetes occurs when your body can't use the insulin naturally produced by the pancreas (called insulin resistance), increasing the risk of heart disease and stroke. Its other tragic side effects include blindness, poor circulation that can lead to amputations, kidney failure, impaired mental function, Alzheimer's disease, and more.

In people with diabetes, excessive blood sugar sticks to the flexible heart muscle like cement through a process known as glycation (AGEs – advanced glycation end products). This results in serious heart problems over time, including heart failure and heart attacks.

The Terrible Trio

Diabetes, obesity, and heart disease are so intimately connected that many doctors treat patients with any of these health issues as though they have all three. This often means they are given 6, 8, 10, or more prescription drugs, each of which has its own side effects requiring more medication to control. It's easy to see that this is a downward spiral that will eventually have fatal consequences.

All of this may seem overwhelming, but it doesn't have to be. Read on and learn how you can overcome all three of these terrible diseases.

French Grape Seed Extract Vanquishes the Terrible Trio – and More

Yes, inflammation is a key underlying cause of obesity, heart disease, stroke, and type 2 diabetes, so it only makes sense that a powerhouse anti-inflammatory like grape seed extract would give the answers we need to vanquish them.

But the FGSE goes much farther than that.

We've said before: We believe that the single most important thing you can do is to follow a healthy eating plan and adopt a healthy lifestyle that includes a moderate amount of exercise, good sleep, and stress management to manage your weight and prevent diabetes. But it is abundantly clear that grape seed extract can help you get back to good health and stay there.

For example, a small, but important pilot study in Thailand found that people who ate a high carbohydrate meal and then took 300 mg of grape seed extract reduced blood sugar levels after a high-carbohydrate meal. The OPCs in grape seed can help stop the roller coaster of high and low blood sugars that lead to insulin resistance and, eventually, to type 2 diabetes.

Important animal studies from France and Spain confirm that overweight hamsters dramatically reduced their waistlines with grape seed extract, even when they were fed a high-fat diet. In addition, the grape seed extract reduced blood sugars, increased the ability to use insulin produced by the pancreas, and lowered blood fats—all important stepping stones to eliminate and prevent heart disease and type 2 diabetes.

Further research confirms that grape seed extract can protect against damage caused by diabetes, including diabetic neuropathy that can lead to amputations.

In an impressive Saudi Arabian study, patients with fatty liver disease, commonly associated with obesity, were given 100 mg of standardized grape seed extract for three months. Their liver function and liver enzyme greatly improved, including severely limiting the number of fat cells that were able to infiltrate the liver. Positive effects were even seen in patients given only 50 mg daily.

And Chinese researchers found that grape seed extract has a powerful antioxidant effect against those dreaded AGEs (advanced glycation end products) that are at least partly responsible for the deadly link between diabetes and heart disease and other complications.

What You Need to Know

- If you have three or more of the following: a fat belly, high blood pressure, high blood sugar, high triglycerides, low HDL cholesterol—you have metabolic syndrome.
- Metabolic syndrome puts you at a very high risk of developing type 2 diabetes and heart disease.
- Obesity is a strong predictor of type 2 diabetes.
- Type 2 diabetes is a strong predictor for all types of heart disease and stroke.
- Grape seed extract reduces belly fat, blood fats, blood pressure, and blood sugar, providing a simple and highly effective answer to these potentially serious health problems.

CHAPTER 9
Stop the Memory Robber

Before we entirely leave the subject of diabetes, it's important to note that Alzheimer's disease has sometimes been called "diabetes of the brain."

Even in the earliest stages of this devastating memory destroying disease, the brain's ability to metabolize sugar is diminished. For decades, science has concluded that the characteristic amyloid plaques and tangles in the brains of Alzheimer's sufferers interrupt the delicate circuitry of thought transmission and memory.

The characteristic beta-amyloid clusters of proteins called "plaques" and clumps of dead and dying nerve and brain cells, called "tangles" are the generally agreed upon indicators that Alzheimer's disease exists.

Think of the brain's network of dendrites and neurons as an electrical system. Those plaques and tangles block the transmission of the electrical current or information through those circuits.

What's the Link?

Many scientists now call Alzheimer's disease "type 3 diabetes." What's the link between Alzheimer's disease and diabetes?

Here are some things that science has proven in recent years that have advanced our understanding of this terrible disease:

- We know that the risk of Alzheimer's disease is doubled in people with diabetes. Some studies say the risk is four-fold higher.
- We also know that the insulin resistance that defines type 2 diabetes, sometimes called "diabesity," is primarily caused by eating too many simple carbs and sugars and not enough fat.
- We also know that insulin resistance starts the brain damage cascade.
- We also know that people with metabolic syndrome are at higher risk of pre-dementia and mild cognitive impairment.
- We also know that diabetes and Alzheimer's disease have parallel underlying causes: impaired insulin signaling, uncontrolled glucose mechanism, oxidative stress, abnormal protein processing, and the stimulation of inflammatory pathways.
- Finally, we know that the increasing and dramatic prevalence of Alzheimer's disease,

diabetes, and obesity have been pretty much in lockstep since 1980.

Does any of this sound familiar? Inflammation? Insulin resistance? Oxidative stress? At least one of these triggers is the underlying cause of virtually every disease discussed in this book. Not surprisingly, French grape seed extract powerfully addresses all of them.

Please re-read Chapter 8 on metabolic syndrome, obesity, and diabetes and apply all of the filters of what you've just learned about Alzheimer's disease to the science laid out here. You'll also see that grape seed extract addresses the underlying causes of cancer, heart disease, and diabetes—and Alzheimer's disease.

Grim Statistics

The Alzheimer's statistics are grim. Alzheimer's disease and dementia cruelly rob the memories of 10% of 65-year-olds, 25% of 75-year-olds, and 50% of 85-year-olds. Alzheimer's disease is now the seventh leading cause of death worldwide, and researchers predict it will affect 106 million people by 2025. By the year 2050, the Alzheimer's Association reports, the number of people 65 and older with Alzheimer's disease will triple.

Patti Reagan, the daughter of President Ronald Reagan, coined the term "The Long Goodbye" in her 2011 book of the same title about her father's lengthy battle against Alzheimer's disease.

Alzheimer's disease victims and their loved ones suffer a long and painful goodbye that takes a terrible toll on families. The average patient lives 10 years or more after diagnosis, growing more and more distant until the body still lives, but the mind is long gone. Only a shell of the loved one remains.

Yes, a small percentage is genetic, but I believe that most Alzheimer's disease is a lifestyle disease, just like diabetes. Control the symptoms of metabolic syndrome, and you not only prevent diabetes and heart disease, but in many cases, you can also prevent Alzheimer's disease.

Alzheimer's disease is considered incurable and irreversible. That may be true, but we'd rather dwell on the idea that Alzheimer's is preventable and that once someone has begun to slide down the slippery slope of memory loss, the deterioration can be slowed or even stopped.

Oxidation and Inflammation

Since the late 1980s, research has hinted that chronic inflammation hastens the Alzheimer's disease process, and there are even some suggestions that inflammation may *cause* Alzheimer's disease.

There is no doubt that inflammation is an important factor in Alzheimer's disease, so it stands to reason that controlling inflammation will reduce the risk of developing the disease.

The same logic applies to oxidative stress from free radical damage.

Free radicals are the culprits in a number of biochemical processes that contribute to Alzheimer's disease, including the formation of advanced glycation end products (AGEs mentioned in Chapter 8), nitration or the constriction of blood vessels because of insufficient nitric oxide, and the accumulation of harmful fats in the bloodstream known as lipid peroxidation.

The above is a pretty fancy way of saying that free radicals certainly play a role in Alzheimer's disease.

Of course, antioxidants neutralize free radicals and even reverse the damage they cause. And you already know from Chapter 1 that French grape seed extract is the most potent antioxidant known to science.

Addressing Alzheimer's Disease and its Underlying Causes

Grape seed OPCs are at the cutting edge of Alzheimer's disease research.

Research shows that grape seed OPCs:

- protect delicate brain circuitry to keep the "electrical" information flowing properly
- reduce the effects of oxidative stress (free radical damage) in the aging brain
- reduce inflammation in the brain
- protect nerve cells to prevent memory loss

- lower blood glucose to protect brain cells

A pivotal 2010 review of Alzheimer's research on grape seed extract from the Mount Sinai School of Medicine shows that grape seed extract (GSE) stops the formation of those beta-amyloid plaques and tangles characteristic of Alzheimer's disease.

Probably the most exciting result of these studies is the confirmation that grape seed extract contributes to brain plasticity, the brain's ability to adapt and create new neural pathways, effectively bypassing obstructions and damaged tissue.

Purdue University researchers noted an interesting pattern: It seems that grape seed extract becomes more effective the longer you take it. The blood and brain levels of catechins and epicatechins, components of OPCs, were detectable as soon as someone took it, but they increased by as much as 282% over time with repeated doses.

Australian researchers found that lab animals given grape seed extract had as much as 44% less brain inflammation and 70% fewer plaques and tangles than animals that did not receive the grape seed OPCs.

The National Center for Complementary and Integrative Health (NCCIH) supports preliminary research on grape seed extract for Alzheimer's disease.

What You Need to Know

- Alzheimer's disease has sometimes been called "diabetes of the brain" or "type 3 diabetes" because of the devastating effect excess blood sugar can have on brain function.
- People with diabetes have at least twice the risk of developing Alzheimer's disease as people with normal blood sugar levels.
- Free radical oxidation and inflammation are important underlying causes of memory loss.
- Grape seed extract OPCs:
    - Protect brain cells, particularly brain cells circuitry
    - Reduce blood sugar
    - Reduce oxidative stress
    - Reduce inflammation
    - Enhance the formation of new neural pathways as alternative circuits for information

CHAPTER 10
A Powerhouse Against Other Diseases and Conditions

If you have read this far, no doubt you are mightily impressed with the considerable healing powers of French grape seed extract.

But there is more. Lots more.

Throughout this book, we've talked about inflammation and oxidation as underlying causes of almost all diseases of aging: cancer, heart disease, diabetes, Alzheimer's disease, and more.

Yes, some of the following diseases and conditions for which grape seed has been proven beneficial are related to inflammation and free radical oxidation—but not all. These are two key considerations in improving overall general health; however, there are some other unique ways that French grape seed extract offers its healing powers.

We're learning more about French grape seed extract's impressive powers against disease and promoting health nearly every day, so a compendium of its benefits will always fall short, but here are some of the best scientifically validated attributes of grape seed.

The body of research on grape seed extract and OPCs has expanded dramatically in recent years, with a total of 2,591 studies on these nutrients listed in the National Library of Medicine's database as of this writing.

Let's look at some of the other ways grape seed extract goes on the offensive against several serious diseases, illnesses, and conditions.

Antibacterial properties: Grape seed extract is a natural antibiotic. Austrian researchers found that GSE killed ten bacterial strains, and other research confirms its effectiveness against antibiotic-resistant *Staph* bacteria that can cause boils, cellulitis, food poisoning, and more. Another study confirms its effectiveness against 343 strains of *Staphylococcus aureus (MRSA)* What's more, Turkish research shows GSE protects kidneys against the damage caused by the prescription antibiotic, amikacin.

Wound healing: Grape seed extract's ability to knock out bacterial infections certainly plays a role in speeding wound healing. Iranian research confirms GSE's healing properties: People who underwent surgeries for the removal of moles or skin tags and given a GSE cream not only had fewer infections but were completely healed in eight days, compared to people who didn't get the grape seed cream, who took 14 days to heal.

Venous insufficiency (leg swelling): This condition is caused by decreased strength and tone in the blood vessel walls that results in swelling, pain, itchiness, and tiredness, usually in the legs. A large Spanish review of studies on the subject confirms that GSE reduces the swelling, pain, cramps, and restless legs associated with the condition.

Healthy eyesight/cataract reduction: The OPCs in grape seed extract are essential for healthy eyesight. They can reduce eyestrain and improve night vision by up to 98% by increasing blood flow to the eyes. OPCs in grape seed extract can also contribute to reducing the size of cataracts. Japanese researchers even found that GSE prevented cataract formation in animals whose heredity made them particularly vulnerable to the condition.

Allergies: As you know, part of the power of OPCs is its anti-inflammatory activity. It turns out that grape seed extract is a natural antihistamine, reducing the sneezing and congestion commonly found in an allergic reaction. This natural antihistamine working with other anti-inflammatory actions can stop allergic reactions, including hives, hay fever, and eczema.

Psoriasis and eczema: Grape seed extract appears to work in a similar way to ease psoriasis inflammation and slow the allergic reactions that cause eczema, both painful and difficult to treat skin conditions.

Attention Deficit/Hyperactivity Disorder (ADHD): A placebo controlled, double-blind study published in the journal *European Child & Adolescent Psychology* found that after just one month, OPCs boosted attention span, caused a significant reduction of hyperactivity and improved motor coordination in children with ADHD. The researchers noted that the symptoms returned one month after stopping the treatment, so OPCs would need to be part of an ongoing regimen. There is conjecture that grape seed extract increases the levels of blood vessel relaxing nitric oxide in the blood, helping increase mental focus. OPCs also regulate the enzymes that produce the brain chemicals dopamine and norepinephrine that help ease the nerve signals of hyperactivity. These findings have great potential for 6.1 million American children with the disorder, 9.4% of children under 18, according to the Centers for Disease Control and Prevention. More are being diagnosed with the disorder at alarming rates, with the numbers expected to increase by 25% in the next five years.

Arthritis: The anti-inflammatory properties of grape seed extract and OPCs significantly ease the pain and swelling of arthritis. But it goes a step farther in rheumatoid arthritis, an autoimmune disease that eventually destroys bones. Korean researchers found that GSE slowed the destruction of bone cells and even stimulated the formation of new bone cells.

Fibromyalgia: The antioxidant and anti-inflammatory powers of grape seed extract help ease this elusive disease's pain and stiffness and protect triggering muscle cells from damage.

Menopause symptoms: Hot flashes, brain fog, mood swings, insomnia, and more characterize the end of a woman's reproductive life. A Japanese study of middle-aged women in the early stages of menopause (perimenopause) showed that the women given either 100 or 200 mg of GSE a day had fewer hot flashes, slept better, had less anxiety and depression, and lower blood pressure. An unexpected bonus: Their lean muscle mass increased in just 8 weeks, meaning they had less fat and better insulin absorption.

Please note that the studies done in the second part of this book were not French grape seed extract. Just imagine how much more powerful the results would be if the superior quality FGSE had been used!

It is clear that grape seed extract targets disease from several directions, some of which we understand well, including inflammation and free radical damage, and others about which we are just learning. There is every reason to predict that the powers of this tiny seed will be even better understood in the coming years.

What You Need to Know

- French grape seed extract mounts a successful offensive against a wide variety of diseases and health conditions beyond its anti-inflammatory and antioxidant effects.
- It has been proven to kill a wide variety of disease-causing bacteria, including *Staphylococcus aureus (MRSA)* and speeds up wound healing.
- It relieves menopause symptoms and increases lean muscle mass in older women, helping them reduce fat and reducing the risk of diabetes.
- It helps children with ADHD to focus better and reduce symptoms of hyperactivity.
- It's a natural antihistamine.
- It relieves eyestrain and prevents cataracts.
- It helps re-build bones in people with rheumatoid arthritis.

CHAPTER 11
Know How to Find the Right Choice

Special insight from Terry:

There is little doubt that French grape seed extract is truly a "gift for health" from nature. If you have cancer or you are at high risk for cancer, you must include FGSE in your daily regimen.

Now here is the caveat in all this: Not all grape seed extracts are created equal. Understanding that there are wildly variable qualities of products available for nearly every botanical and supplement is a key part of understanding why some products are exceptionally effective when taken in the correct dosages, and others are utterly without effect. Unlike pharmaceuticals, where the drug prescribed is exactly the same as the drug dispensed, this is often not the case in the nutritional supplements industry.

Just pause a moment here to think about our uniqueness as humans. Plants have their own uniqueness, called bioindividuality. Their medicinal powers vary due to the climate, the level of water, sunshine or shade, and the proper time to harvest. For example, plants harvested in the morning may yield a totally different level of natural compounds than plants harvested late in the day.

There are numerous grape seed products available that vary greatly in quality and price point.

Yes, you can buy "grape seed extract" for as little as 12 cents a serving. In this case, cheaper is absolutely not better. Your money can be washing right down the drain.

These inexpensive brands are made from a cheap Chinese grape seed extract that is minimally absorbable and has few, if any, of the beneficial compounds and health benefits attributed to this natural botanical in hundreds of published studies. Any extract that originates from grape seeds is considered "grape seed extract", but that is where the similarity ends.

Now, we're not saying that the most expensive brands of supplements are always the best. But in this case, yes, it is well worth spending a little more—about 40 cents a serving—to ensure that the product actually contains the nutrients that your body needs to use the healing power of this powerful and well-studied nutrient.

What's the Difference?

First of all, absorbability is essential to any type of supplement. Whatever the nutrient in question, if your body can't use it, you're quite literally flushing your money down the toilet. Scientifically, that's called bioavailability.

Without question, you always want the most bioavailable products possible.

French grape seed extract comes from grapes grown in France's wine regions, where some of the world's finest wines are produced. They are rich sources of polyphenols, abundant plant nutrients that are the underlying source of protection against all of the diseases we've examined in this book.

The ideal French grape seed extract is free of tannins. While those tannins give wines their body and flavor, they are not absorbable, so they don't provide any health benefits. You don't want them in your grape seed extract.

The OPCs in other forms of grape seed extract typically are composed of a variety of weights and sizes. The large non-absorbable molecules in grape seed extract are known as condensed tannins, which have no health benefits and are not absorbed by the human body.

Cheaper forms of grape seed extract are often spiked with additional tannins intended to bulk them up, resulting in low prices and fewer health benefits since they cannot be used by the human body.

Look for a tannin-free product with a small molecular structure for maximum absorption which has 99% polyphenols, 80% OPCs, and 27-32% dimers.

If that sounds like a complicated search, let me reassure you that it's not complicated at all.

One-Two Punch

French grape seed extract is unquestionably one of the most formidable foes of cancer and other chronic diseases.

Now we have the greatest combination of botanical cancer fighters known to modern science: French grape seed extract and curcumin . Together, this combo attacks cancer in more ways than any other single botanical or pharmaceutical with more success.

Curcumin is a highly studied botanical with proven effects against all of the diseases of aging, including cancer.

Knowing the powerful anti-cancer properties of French grape seed extract piqued my curiosity. What if we combined French grape seed extract with curcumin?

Why curcumin? A few years back, Dr. Goel's team researched the anti-cancer properties of curcumin on cancer, with especially important findings showing curcumin's impressive anti-cancer effect and its abilities to kill cancer stem cells.

Combining French grape seed extract VX1 and curcumin, the two became an unbeatable cancer-fighting team. You've no doubt heard the word "synergy," which means the whole is greater than the sum of the parts. In this case, putting FGSE and curcumin together attack cancer more powerfully than science predicts.

I can only imagine how much future findings will prove the combined power of curcumin and French grape seed OPCs to prevent, treat, and even cure cancer.

I'm impressed with other research that confirms the power of curcumin.

In 2012, a randomized pilot study was carried out to assess the effectiveness and safety of curcumin in patients with active rheumatoid arthritis. The results showed better benefits in the patients taking curcumin than those taking the anti-inflammatory pharmaceutical, diclofenac (sold under the brand names Voltaren and others). This is remarkable since, unlike diclofenac, curcumin has no side effects.

Another study published in *Phytotherapy Research* in 2016 showed curcumin's positive outcomes in reducing the symptoms of depression and even surpasses some of the most commonly used anti-depressants.

There are numerous other studies done or in progress or planned all over the world on Alzheimer's disease, various types of cancers, heart disease, diabetes, and many others.

Botanical supplements are made up of hundreds of molecules that work on multiple pathways in the body at multiple levels of those pathways, all simultaneously. It's like having a pharmacy in a bottle without the fear of side effects. Drugs are limited to what they can accomplish as they are only made up of one molecule targeting one pathway in the body, therefore, throwing many other pathways out of balance, and the benefits are limited as well.

In my experience, these natural ingredients can have impressive long-term benefits. They are free from the side effects and complications caused by pharmaceuticals.

Dosage

Here is a list of recommended dosages for conditions French grape seed extract VX1 can address. Obviously, you should always be under the care of a physician and/or a holistically-oriented physician with a background and an understanding of scientifically-validated nutritional ingredients.

Cancer support:	400-1200 mg daily
Help in supporting cancer prevention:	150-400 mg daily
Support optimal blood pressure:	150-300 mg daily
Support cardiovascular health:	300-600 mg daily
Alzheimer's disease:	300-600 mg daily
Support veins in legs:	150-300 mg daily

A Combo?

An obvious combination would be OPCs with curcumin. Wouldn't this make a phenomenal daily supplement to prevent and treat cancer? Just looking at the ORAC antioxidant power of these two ingredients is remarkable, with curcumin hitting 1.5 million per 100 grams while French grape seed extract comes in at 2 million per 100 grams—Wow! That is unparalleled antioxidant power! We know that free radical oxygen molecules lead to imperfect cell reproduction, so that alone should be an incentive to nip cancer in the bud.

There is also a possible 3-4 punch to combine with the 1-2 punch against cancer: Boswellia, a well-researched anti-inflammatory herb, also known as frankincense, and andrographis, an Ayurvedic herb. Current research suggests the two can add even more power to the anti-cancer regimen.

CHAPTER 12
Doc to Doc

Dear Reader,

We all know our doctors and other health care professionals are very busy. As excited as you may be about this book and all it offers, it's unlikely you can persuade a medical professional to read the entire book. That's why we have written this information-packed and very concise summary of the contents of this book specifically for people with scientific backgrounds. Most authors jealously protect their copyrights, but in this case, we encourage you to photocopy, scan, or photograph the pages in this chapter and distribute them freely to health care professionals.

From Dr. Goel:

Dear Health Care Professional,

Your patient has given you a copy of this chapter with our blessings and permission. We have given it to the public domain so that the vital information it contains on the value of French grape seed extract oligomeric proanthocyanidins (OPCs) in prevention, treatment, and eradication of cancer can be widely distributed.

My 20 years of research as Director of Epigenetics and Cancer Prevention at Baylor University Medical Center in Dallas and my current position as Professor and Chair, Department of Molecular Diagnostics, Therapeutics and Translational Oncology at City of Hope in Duarte, CA have largely focused on gastrointestinal cancers. I submit that these findings apply to many, perhaps most, other forms of cancer.

This book is written primarily about the effects of French grape seed extract OPCs. I also endorse a combination therapy with a particular form of curcumin, as confirmed in my research. In addition, the book contains important information on the positive effects of OPCs against other chronic diseases of aging.

I understand that doctors are frequently skeptical about natural formulations and, if they haven't conducted their own research investigations on a subject, they are inclined to steer their patients away from them, even though these formulations might be lifesaving. I urge you to spend a few minutes reviewing these findings. Confirm them for yourself, and consider adding them to your cancer protocols.

In brief, this is what we've learned about a specific formulation of tannin-free French grape seed OPCs and their unique multi-directional approaches to cancer cells:

- Inhibit inflammation
- Antioxidant
- Inhibit carcinogenesis
- Induce apoptosis
- Inhibit angiogenesis
- Neutralize free radical oxygen molecules
- Inhibit the pathways that form and support formation of cancer stem cells
- Overcome chemoresistance
- Work synergistically with conventional chemotherapy pharmaceuticals, enhancing their effectiveness
- Chemoprotective
- Inhibit metastasis
- Safe and non-toxic even when taken in large amounts

French grape seed extract OPCs have been well researched and well validated for their anti-inflammatory and antioxidant properties. In fact, an ORAC value for French grape seed extract has not been established because it exceeds measuring capability parameters at 150,000 per gram.

Let's look a little farther into the findings on three pivotal studies conducted by my research team:

Carcinogenesis

A study from my team published in 2018 in the journal *Carcinogenesis,* showed that OPCs halted communication in all six known cancer cell-forming pathways.

Cancer Stem Cells

In our study published in *Scientific Reports* 2018, we created organoids from current colorectal cancer patients to test the effects of OPCs on cancer stem cells. The OPCs in French grape seed extract *killed* cancer stem cells. French grape seed extract is the *only* substance, natural or chemical, other than curcumin that stops cancer stem cells from reproducing.

In addition to finding that OPCs inhibited cancer stem cell reproduction, our team found that those OPCs prevented all forms of carcinogenesis, tumorigenesis, and angiogenesis and induced apoptosis.

Multifaceted Signaling

In the 2018 study published in *Carcinogenesis*, my team found that the smaller OPC molecules in French grape seed extract were able to lock down cancer cells and stop them from forming tumors. Those OPCs were also able to alter genes involved in cell cycle and DNA replication across multiple cell lines. In addition, OPCs directly engaged multiple signaling pathways, suppressing cellular expression, inhibiting angiogenesis, inducing apoptosis, and promoting homeostasis.

Chemoresistance

Our OPC research published in *Carcinogenesis* in 2019 provides the hope that so many cancer patients seek in the face of nearly inevitable chemoresistance.

Not only does the OPC combo from French grape seed extract break down the ABC pathway firewall, reducing tumor growth within mere *hours*, it also sensitizes the cancer cells to the impact of conventional chemotherapy drugs. Therefore the patient needs fewer drugs and experiences fewer side effects.

Combination Therapy

Our additional 2018 work, published in *Scientific Reports*, validated the efficacy of a combination of French grape seed extract and curcumin, demonstrating superior anti-tumorigenic properties.

There are no pharmaceuticals that have these properties, largely because conventional anti-cancer drugs throw RNA sequences out of balance. They further disrupt homeostasis and require other drugs to try to bring the body back in balance, creating a vicious circle and a downward spiral that I am certain you have witnessed in your patients.

Like you, I am a scientist, not at all given to hyperbole, but I am deeply encouraged by the magnitude of these findings. They are already changing the way we treat our patients, even those with late-stage cancers, changing their chances of survival and offering them a vastly improved quality of life.

Other Chronic Diseases of Aging
In addition to their considerable anti-cancer properties, OPCs have been extensively researched for their efficacy against various other diseases and health conditions.

Among them:

Cardiovascular disease
- Anti-hypertensive
- Vasodilator
- Reduces oxidized LDL cholesterol and blood triglycerides
- Protective against fatty liver disease
- Anti-coagulant
- Addresses metabolic syndrome

Diabetes and obesity
- Reduced blood glucose
- Improved insulin resistance
- Reduces belly fat
- Inhibits Advanced Glycation End products that are implicated in diseases of aging

Alzheimer's disease
- Reduces oxidative stress and inflammation in brain tissues
- Neuroprotective
- Reduced blood glucose is neuroprotective

Additionally, French grape seed extract OPCs have been shown to:

- Have substantial antibacterial activities, even against resistant MRSA
- Promote wound healing
- Address venous insufficiency and restless leg syndrome
- Inhibit cataract formation and improve night vision
- Anti-allergenic and antihistaminic
- Reduce inflammation and flares of eczema and psoriasis
- Improve attention span and motor coordination in patients with ADHD
- Reduce symptoms of menopause

All OPCs Are Not Created Equal

Bioavailability is essential to the efficacy of any treatment. The best French grape seed extract product should be tannin-free since tannins inhibit absorption. Small molecular structure is also important to bioavailability.

In my opinion, the best FSGE product is a formulation that has 99% polyphenols, 80% OPCs, and 27-32% dimers.

The recommended dosage for patients with active cancers is 400 to 1200 mg daily. There have been no documented side effects.

Bioavailabilty is also an issue with curcumin products. I highly recommend adding a curcumin with turmeric essential oil for its validated bioavailability because of proprietary extraction techniques and its synergistic effects when used with French grape seed extract. Optimal dosage for patients with advanced cancers should be 1200-3000 mg daily. No side effects have been documented at these dosages.

Dosages from 100-300 mg daily are effective for other conditions.

Finally…

Natural products are made up of hundreds of molecules that work on multiple pathways in the body at multiple levels of those pathways, all simultaneously. Botanicals are like having a pharmacy in a bottle without the fear of side effects. Pharmaceuticals, especially those that target cancer in various ways, are limited to what they can accomplish. They are composed of one molecule targeting one pathway in the body, therefore, throwing many other pathways out of balance, and the benefits are limited as well.

In my experience, these natural ingredients can have impressive long-term benefits. They are free from the side effects and complications caused by pharmaceuticals. More and more physicians are beginning to see that the side effects of drugs often outweigh their benefits.

I enthusiastically support the use of French grape seed extract OPCs to prevent, treat, and reverse cancers and the other diseases mentioned in this chapter.

Health care professionals who would like to discuss these findings with me are welcome to contact me through my publisher, Terry Talks Nutrition Publishing:

info@ttnpublishing.com

Thanks for your attention,
Ajay Goel, Ph.D.
Duarte, CA

References

The most recent publications on French grape seed extract OPCs from Dr. Goel's Team:

Ravindranathan P, Pasham D, Balaji U, Goel A et al; Mechanistic insights into anticancer properties of oligomeric proanthocyanidins from grape seeds in colorectal cancer. Carcinogenesis. 2018 May 28;39(6):767-777.

Ravindranathan P, Pasham D, Goel A. Oligomeric proanthocyanidins (OPCs) from grape seed extract suppress the activity of ABC transporters in overcoming chemoresistance in colorectal cancer cells. Carcinogenesis. 2019 May 14;40(3):412-421.

Toden S, Ravindranathan P, Gu J, Goel A et al. Oligomeric proanthocyanidins (OPCs) target cancer stem-like cells and suppress tumor organoid formation in colorectal cancer. *Scientific Reports.* 2018 Feb 20;8(1):3335.

Ravindranathan P, Pasham D, Balaji U et al. A combination of curcumin and oligomeric proanthycyanidins offer superior anti-tumorigenic properties in colorectal cancer. *Scientific Reports.* 2018 Sep 14;8(1):13869.

About the Authors

Terry Lemerond

Terry Lemerond is a natural health expert with over 50 years of experience helping people live healthier, happier lives. A much sought-after speaker and accomplished author, Terry shares his wealth of experience and knowledge in health and nutrition through his educational programs, including the Terry Talks Nutrition website—TerryTalksNutrition.com—newsletters, podcasts, webinars, and personal speaking engagements. Terry has also hosted Terry Talks Nutrition radio for the past 30 years. His books include *Seven Keys to Vibrant Health*, *Seven Keys to Unlimited Personal Achievement*, and *50+ Natural Health Secrets Proven to Change Your Life.* Terry continues to author and co-author books to educate everyone on the steps they can take to live a more healthy vibrant life.

His continual dedication, energy, and zeal are part of his ongoing mission—to help everyone improve their health.

Dr. Ajay Goel

Dynamic and passionate—with a formidable record of patented innovations in cancer care—Ajay Goel, Ph.D., M.S., is committed to developing better methods for the early detection and precision treatment of cancer.

He joined City of Hope in June 2019 as founding chair of the new Department of Molecular Diagnostics and Experimental Therapeutics and founding director of Biotech Innovations at Beckman Research Institute.

A noted expert in gastrointestinal and other cancers, Dr. Goel is currently developing early-detection blood tests for colon, pancreatic and ovarian cancers and a test for pancreatic cancer that can detect the disease seven years earlier than is now possible. Within the next few years, these tests are expected to become a simple and affordable part of everyone's annual health physical, just like diabetes or cholesterol tests. He is also working with genomic-based precision oncology to answer the question: Why do therapies work with some good candidates and not with others?

Dr. Goel was born in India, received his Ph. D. in biophysics from Punjab University, completed his postgraduate work at the University of California, San Diego, and went on to a noteworthy 16-year career at Baylor Scott & White Research Institute in Texas. He has authored more than 300 articles in peer-reviewed international journals and holds more than 30 advanced genomic and transcriptomic international patents.

References

PART 1
French Grape Seed Extract and Cancer

Chapter 1: Introducing a Powerhouse Botanical

ORAC table download:
www.ars.usda.gov/nutrientdata/ORAC

Sinclair DA. Toward a unified theory of caloric restriction and longevity regulation. *Mechanics of Ageing and Development*. 2005 Sep;126(9):987-1002.

Baur JA, Pearson KJ, Price NL, et al. Resveratrol improves health and survival of mice on a high-calorie diet. *Nature*. 2006 Nov 16;444(7117):337-42.

Bhullar KS, Hubbard BP. Lifespan and health span extension by resveratrol.

Biochim Biophys Acta. 2015 Jun;1852(6):1209-18.

Chapter 2: A Powerful Natural Answer to Cancer

World Health Organization cancer data: https://www.who.int/cancer/PRGlobocanFinal.pdf

Narod SA, JavaidIqbal, Miller AB. Why have breast cancer mortality rates declined? *Journal of Cancer Policy.* Volume 5, September 2015, Pages 8-17

Toden S, Goel A. Novel and previously unknown mechanisms of action by which low molecular weight oligomeric proanthocyanins (OPC) from French Grape Seed Extract VX1 help eradicate colorectal cancer cells. Oligomeric proanthocyanidins inhibit Hippo-YAP pathway and prevent colorectal cancer stem cell formation. Poster presentation at the annual American Association for Cancer Research (AACR) meeting. New Orleans, LA. April 16-20, 2016.

Mao JT, Xue B et al. MicroRNA-19a/b mediates grape seed procyanidin extract-induced anti-neoplastic effects against lung cancer. *Journal of Nutritional Biochemistry.* 2016 May 20;34:118-125.

Scrobata I, Bolfa P et al. Natural chemopreventive alternatives in oral cancer chemoprevention. *Journal of Physiology and Pharmacology; 2*016 Feb;67(1):161-72.

Derry M, Raina K et al. Differential effects of grape seed extract against human colorectal cancer cell lines: The intricate role of death receptors and mitochondria. *Cancer Letters.* 2012 Dec 23.

Sharma G, Tyagi AK et al. Synergistic anti-cancer effects of grape seed extract and conventional cytotoxic agent doxorubicin against human breast carcinoma cells. *Breast Cancer Research and Treatment;* 2004 May;85(1):1-12.

Sharma SD, Meeran Sm et al. Proanthocyanidins inhibit in vitro and in vivo growth of human non-small cell lung cancer cells by inhibiting the prostaglandin E(2) and prostaglandin E(2) receptors. *Molecular Cancer Therapy;* 2010 Mar;9(3):569-80.

Dinicola S, Cucina A et al. Apoptosis-inducing factor and caspase-dependent apoptotic pathways triggered by different grape seed extracts on human colon cancer cell line Caco-2. *British Journal of Nutrition;* 2010 Sep;104(6):824-32.

Chao C, Slezak JM et al. Alcoholic beverage intake and risk of lung cancer: the California Men's Health Study. *Cancer Epidemiology,Biomarkers and Prevention;* 2008 Oct;17(10):2692-9.

Chapter 3: A Shotgun Approach to Cancer

Ravindranathan P, Pasham D, Balaji U et al; Mechanistic insights into anticancer properties of oligomeric proanthocyanidins from grape seeds in colorectal cancer. *Carcinogenesis* , 2018. -1-11.

Ravindranathan P, Pasham D, Goel A. Oligomeric proanthocyanidins (OPCs) from grape seed extract suppress the activity of ABC transporters in overcoming chemoresistance in colorectal cancer cells. *Carcinogenesis* 2019. P. 1-10.

Chapter 4: Wipe Out Cancer Stem Cells

Toden S, Ravindranathan P, Gu J et al. Oligomeric proanthocyanidins (OPCs) target cancer stem-like cells and suppress tumor organoid formation in colorectal cancer. *Scientific Reports*. Published online 20 February 2018.

Chapter 5: The One-Two Punch

Ravindranathan P, Pasham D, Balaji U et al. A combination of curcumin and oligomeric proanthycyanidins offer superior anti-tumorigenic properties in colorectal cancer. *Scientific Reports* 2018 Sep 14;8(1):13869.

REFERENCES

PART 2:
French Grape Seed Extract and Other Diseases

Chapter 6: Insidious Inflammation and Obdurate Oxidation

Cohen S, Janick-Deverts D et al. Chronic Stress, glucocortisoid receptor resistance, inflammation and disease risk. *Proceedings of the National Academy of Sciences USA.* 2012 Apr 17;109(16):5995-9. doi: 10.1073/pnas.1118355109.

Facino RM, et all. Free radicals scavenging action and anti-enzyme activities of Proanthocyanadins from Vitis vinifera. *Arzneim Forsch*, 1994; 44: 592–601.

Terra, X, Valls, J et al. Grape-Seed Procyanidins Act as Anti-inflammatory Agents in Endotoxin-Stimulated RAW 264.7 Macrophages by Inhibiting NFkB Signaling Pathway. *Journal of Agricultural and Food Chemistry*; 4357-4365.

Das, S, Das, D. Anti-Inflammatory Responses of Resveratrol. *Inflammation & Allergy-Drug Targets IADT* 2007; 168-173.

Chapter 7: A Guardian Against Heart Disease

Hertog MG, Feskens EJ et al. Dietary antioxidant flavonoids and risk of coronary heart disease: the Zutphen Elderly Study. *Lancet;* 1993 Oct 23;342(8878):1007-11.

Belcaro G et al. Grape seed procyanidins in pre- and mild hypertension: a registry study. *Evidence-Based Complementary and Alternative Med;* 2013;2013:313142.

Carlson S, Peng N et al. The effects of botanical dietary supplements on cardiovascular, cognitive and metabolic function in males and females. *Gender Medicine;* 2008; 5(SuppA);S76-S90.

Park E, Edirisinsghe I et al. Effects of grape seed extract beverage on blood pressure and metabolic indices in individuals with pre-hypertension: a randomised, double-blinded, two-arm, parallel, placebo-controlled trial. *British Journal of Nutrition;* 2016 Jan 28;115(2):226-38

Fitzpatrick DF et al. Vasodilating procyanidins derived from grape seeds. *Annals of the New York Academy of Sciences;* 2002; 957:78-89. *LoS One;* 2015 Oct 12;10(10):e0140267.

Downing LE, Heidker RM et al. A Grape Seed Procyanidin Extract Ameliorates Fructose-Induced Hypertriglyceridemia in Rats via Enhanced Fecal Bile

Acid and Cholesterol Excretion and Inhibition of Hepatic Lipogenesis. *Los One;* 2015 Oct 12;10(10):e0140267.

Preuss HG, Wallerstedt D et al. Effects of niacin-bound chromium and grape seed proanthocyanidin extract on the lipid profile of hypercholesterolemic subjects: a pilot study. *Journal of Medicine*; 2000;31(5-6):227-46.

Sano T, Oda E et al. Anti-thrombotic effect of proanthocyanidin, a purified ingredient of grape seed. *Thrombosis Research;* 2005;115(1-2):115-21.

Chapter 8: Metabolic diseases, obesity and diabetes

Ardid-Ruiz A, Harazin A, Bama L et al. The effects of Vitis vinifera L. phenolic compounds on a blood-brain barrier culture model: Expression of leptin receptors and protection against cytokine-induced damage. J Ethnopharmacol. 2020 Jan 30;247:112253.

Aguilar M, Bhuket T et al. Prevalence of the metabolic syndrome in the United States, 2003-2012. *Journal of the American Medical Association;2015;* May 19;313(19):1973-4.

Sung, KC, Rhee EJ et al. Increased Cardiovascular Mortality in Subjects With Metabolic Syndrome Is Largely Attributable to Diabetes and Hypertension in 159,971 Korean Adults. *Journal of Clinical Endocrinology and Metabolism;* 2015 Jul;100(7):2606-12.

Ogden, CL, Carroll MD et al. Prevalence of Overweight and Obesity in the United States, 1999-2004. *Journal of the American Medical Association;* 2006;295(13):1549-1555.

Sapwarobol S, et al. Postprandial blood glucose response to grape seed extract in healthy participants: A pilot study. *Pharmacogn Mag.* 2012;8(31):192-6. *Pharmacognosy Magazine;* 2012 Jul;8(31):192-6.

[Baskaran Yogalakshmi, Saravanan Bhuvaneswari, S Sreeja, Carani Venkatraman Anuradha.](#) Grape seed proanthocyanidins and metformin act by different mechanisms to promote insulin signaling in rats fed high calorie diet. [*Journal of Cell Communication and Signaling;* 2013 Sep 12.](#)

Caimari A, del Bas JM et al. Low doses of grape seed procyanidins reduce adiposity and improve the plasma lipid profile in hamsters. International Journal, of Obesity (London);2013 Apr;37(4):576-83.

Chapter 9: Stop the Memory Robber

Campos-Pena V, Toral-Rios D et al. Metabolic syndrome as a risk factor for Alzheimer's disease: is Aβ a crucial factor in both pathologies? *Antioxidants and Redox Signaling;* 2016 Jul 1.

REFERENCES

Rani V, Deshmukh R et al. Alzheimer's disease: Is this a brain specific diabetic condition? *Physiology and Behavior;* 2016 May 25;164(Pt A):259-267.

Wang J, Bi W et al. Targeting multiple pathogenic mechanisms with polyphenols for the treatment of Alzheimer's disease-experimental approach and therapeutic implications. *Frontiers in Aging Neuroscience;* 2014 Mar 14;6:42.

Perry G, Cash A et al. Alzheimer Disease and Oxidative Stress. *Journal of Biomedicine and Biotechnology*; 2002;2(3):120-123.

Pasinetti G, Ho L. Role of grape seed polyphenols in Alzheimer's disease neuropathology. *Nutrition and Dietary Supplements*; 2010 Aug 1; 2010(2): 97–103.

Wang YJ, Thomas P et al. Consumption of grape seed extract prevents amyloid-beta deposition and attenuates inflammation in brain of an Alzheimer's disease mouse. *Neurotoxicology Research;* 2009 Jan;15(1):3-14.

Feruzzi MG, Lobo JK et al. Bioavailability of gallic acid and catechins from grape seed polyphenol extract is improved by repeated dosing in rats: implications for treatment in Alzheimer's disease. *Journal of Alzheimer's Disease*; 2009;18(1):113-24

Chapter 10: A Powerhouse Against Other Diseases and Conditions

Mayer R et al. Proanthocyanidins: target compounds as antibacterial agents. *Journal of Agriculture and Food Chemistry*; 2008;56(16):6959-66.

Al-Habib A, et al. Bactericidal effect of grape seed extract on methicillin-resistant Staphylococcus aureus (MRSA). *Journal of Toxicological Sciences;* 2010;35(3):357-64.

Hemmati AA, Foroozan M et al. The topical effect of grape seed extract 2% cream on surgery wound healing. *Global Journal of Health Science;* 2014 Oct 29;7(3):52-8.

Martinez-Zapata MJ, Vernooii RW et al. Phlebotonics for venous insufficiency. *Cochrane Database of Systematic Reviews*; 2016 Apr 6;4:CD003229.

More about TTN Publishing, LLC

Everyone has the same desire: a vibrant, healthy life!

TTN Publishing exists to provide educational information anyone can use to understand how herbs and botanical medicines play a vital role in optimal health. From a stomach ache to a life-threatening disease, even cancer, the plant kingdom has safe, effective phytonutrients and answers for healthy living.

Author and health pioneer Terry Lemerond brings his vast knowledge of plant medicines combined with cutting edge research from today's top scientists and doctors directly to consumers. Each TTN Publishing, LLC book is crafted to provide the necessary basic information and recommendations for how botanicals can be used in practical ways to fight disease and improve the path to healthy living.

Education, information, scientific validation, and common sense are a part of every TTN Publishing endeavor. There are many books to come, so stay connected! With 80 percent of the world's population depending on plant medicines, you can join in the knowledge and wisdom available to meet your health goals.

Welcome to TTN Publishing!

We'd love to hear from you!
info@ttnpublishing.com
www.TTNPublishing.com
Would you like to be one of the first to know the latest updates on Terry's books?

- Learn more about his background and new books
- See photos, videos, and the latest news
- Listen to Terry's radio show, including archived programs on a multitude of subjects
- Sign up for a free weekly email newsletter and educational webinar notices

It's all available at TerryTalksNutrition.com

Don't forget to connect at:
www.facebook.com/TerryTalksNutrition

Share this exciting news!

If you appreciated this book, please let others know.

- Pick up another copy and share with a friend
- Talk about it on social media
- Write a review on your blog or website
- Recommend this book to friends and family

Thank you for being a true health seeker!
TTN Publishing, LLC

Printed in Great Britain
by Amazon